# Antibiotics and Their Mechanisms of Action

AF890331

Deepesh Nagarajan
Editor

# Antibiotics and Their Mechanisms of Action

Springer

*Editor*
Deepesh Nagarajan
Biotechnology
Ramaiah University of Applied Sciences
Bangalore, Karnataka, India

ISBN 978-981-97-6853-0 ISBN 978-981-97-6851-6 (eBook)
https://doi.org/10.1007/978-981-97-6851-6

© The Editor(s) (if applicable) and The Author(s), under exclusive license to Springer Nature Singapore Pte Ltd. 2024

This work is subject to copyright. All rights are solely and exclusively licensed by the Publisher, whether the whole or part of the material is concerned, specifically the rights of translation, reprinting, reuse of illustrations, recitation, broadcasting, reproduction on microfilms or in any other physical way, and transmission or information storage and retrieval, electronic adaptation, computer software, or by similar or dissimilar methodology now known or hereafter developed.
The use of general descriptive names, registered names, trademarks, service marks, etc. in this publication does not imply, even in the absence of a specific statement, that such names are exempt from the relevant protective laws and regulations and therefore free for general use.
The publisher, the authors and the editors are safe to assume that the advice and information in this book are believed to be true and accurate at the date of publication. Neither the publisher nor the authors or the editors give a warranty, expressed or implied, with respect to the material contained herein or for any errors or omissions that may have been made. The publisher remains neutral with regard to jurisdictional claims in published maps and institutional affiliations.

This Springer imprint is published by the registered company Springer Nature Singapore Pte Ltd.
The registered company address is: 152 Beach Road, #21-01/04 Gateway East, Singapore 189721, Singapore

If disposing of this product, please recycle the paper.

*This book is dedicated to my grandfathers.*

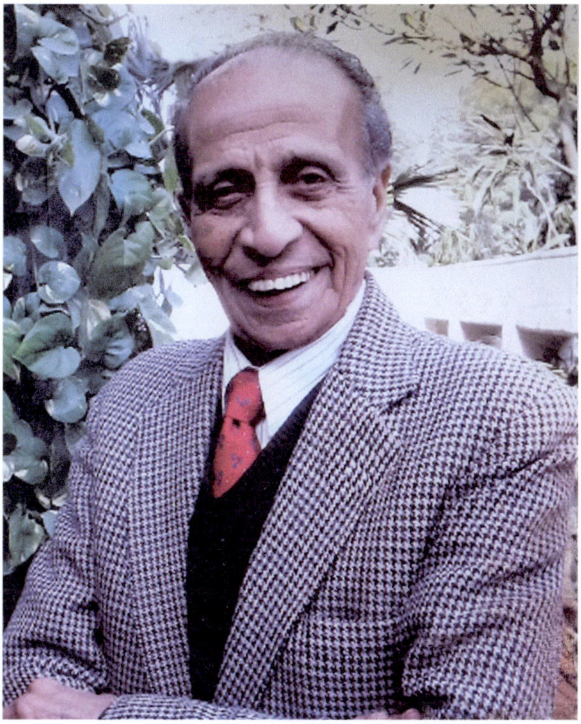

**Dr. Shankaran Krishnamurthy**
**(1925-2005)**

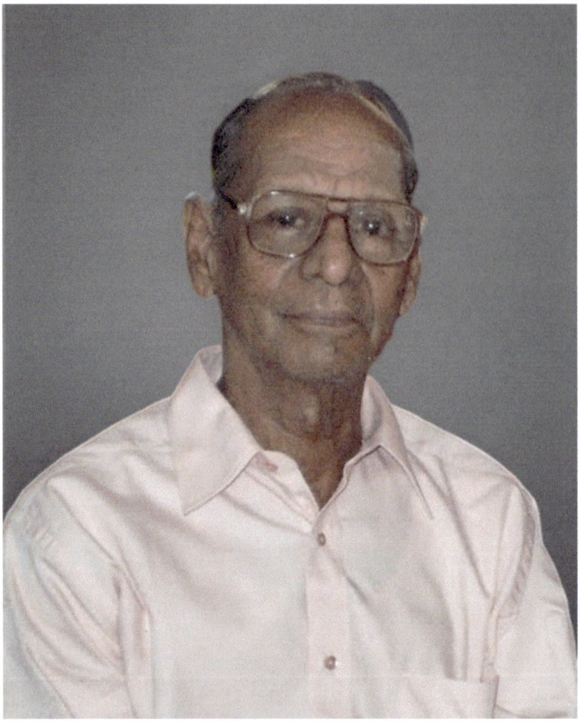

**Krishnamurthy Subramanian**
**(1924-2022)**

# Preface

Any undergraduate student studying microbiology in any university in any country will eventually have to take a course on antibiotics. When undergraduates are taught this topic, a strong emphasis is always placed on their use from the clinician's perspective. What diseases is rifampicin used to treat? What substances should be co-administered alongside amoxicillin to inhibit bacterial $\beta$-lactamases? What is a drug of last resort, and why is it called so? These pressing questions are all rightly answered in any textbook on antibiotics (including this one).

While a textbook with a strong clinical emphasis is required to train the future doctor, it does a disservice to the future scientist. How are antibiotics discovered? How are their mechanisms of action elucidated? How do I pick the right experiment for the right problem? These are all questions a research-oriented undergraduate must not just know the answers to, but must be equipped to address in the laboratory when staring at a small aliquot of strange white powder in a centrifuge tube that *may* possess some antimicrobial properties.

*Antibiotics and Their Mechanisms of Action* attempts to do just that. Rather than merely state "penicillin inhibits cell wall synthesis," this textbook will explain every observation and experiment that backed this conclusion, and will do so for the mechanism of action for every class of antibiotics discussed.

I completed my bachelors in 2010 before joining the Indian Institute of Science for what I consider to be the most productive time of my life. My PhD involved designing and testing new antibiotic candidates, a task that my undergraduate and even postgraduate theory classes scarcely prepared me for. This textbook was written for you: the student and future researcher. You have a world-class intellect. You are capable of joining the very best research programs the world has to offer. You have an exciting career ahead, and you should only expect your education to prepare you for it.

Bangalore, India
Mumbai, India

Deepesh Nagarajan

# Contents

# About the Authors

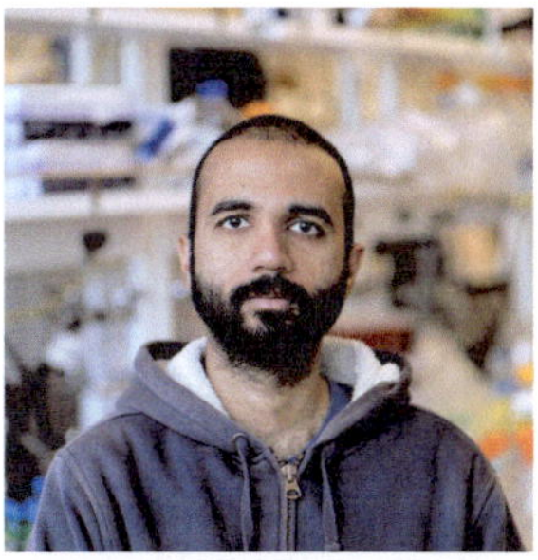

**Dr. Deepesh Nagarajan** completed his PhD in 2017 at the Indian Institute of Science, Bangalore, in the field of protein design. He completed a post-doctoral fellowship at the University of Washington under Prof. David Baker, who is the leading protein designer in the field. Dr. Nagarajan is interested in the applications of protein design approaches to drug development, and has had a decade of experience designing antimicrobial peptides.

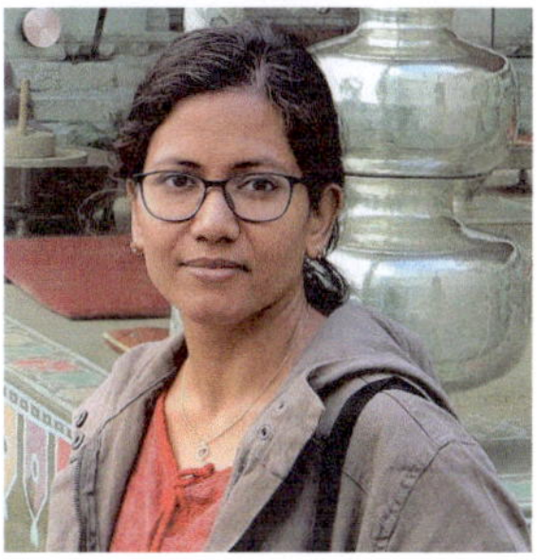

**Dr. Pampi Chakraborty** has been teaching in the Department of Microbiology, St. Xavier's College, Mumbai, since 2014. After finishing her MSc in Microbiology from Calcutta University, she joined Bhabha Atomic Research Centre, Mumbai, in 2006 for her PhD. Her thesis was entitled "Host-pathogen interactions of different strains of Mycobacterium tuberculosis" and was submitted to the Homi Bhabha National Institute. She teaches molecular biology, immunology, and genetics to undergraduate and postgraduate students. She has also mentored some research students.

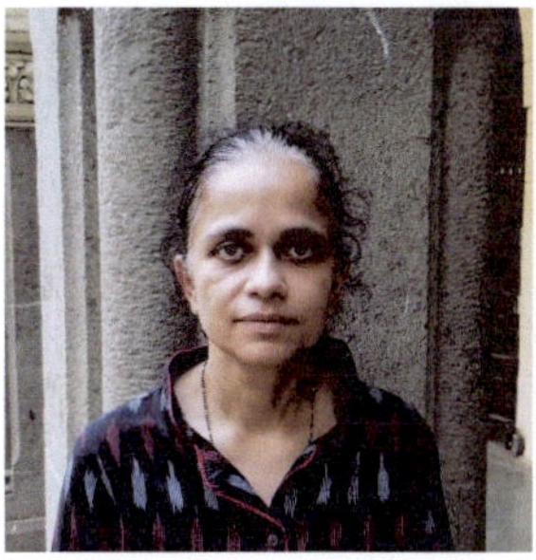

**Dr. Aparna Shetye** completed her PhD in virology from the Weill Cornell Graduate School of Medical Sciences. She worked on the mechanisms of entry of the Measles and Nipah viruses in order to elucidate commonalities in the entry of paramyxoviruses. She has been working as an assistant professor since 2013 at the Department of Microbiology, St Xavier's College, Mumbai. She teaches virology, biochemistry, and biostatistics to both undergraduate and postgraduate students. Her interests include viral entry and environmental microbiology.

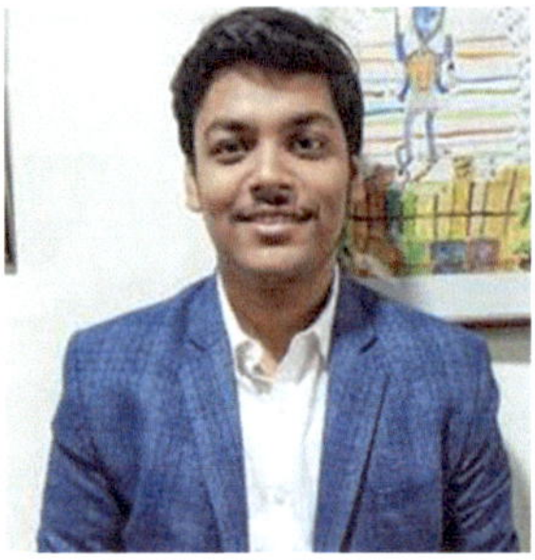

**Subhrojyoti Ghosh** is an MTech student at the Indian Institute of Technology, Madras, in the field of Bioprocess Engineering. He is also a course instructor at Udemy and lectures on a YouTube Channel named "Biotech Basics." He has worked earlier on identifying potential biological agents triggering Epstein-Barr Virus (EBV) Reactivation in association with the Indian Institute of Technology Indore. Presently, he studies the role of motility on microbial chemotaxis and has diversified research interests, including antimicrobial resistance, drug development, chemotaxis, and metastasis.

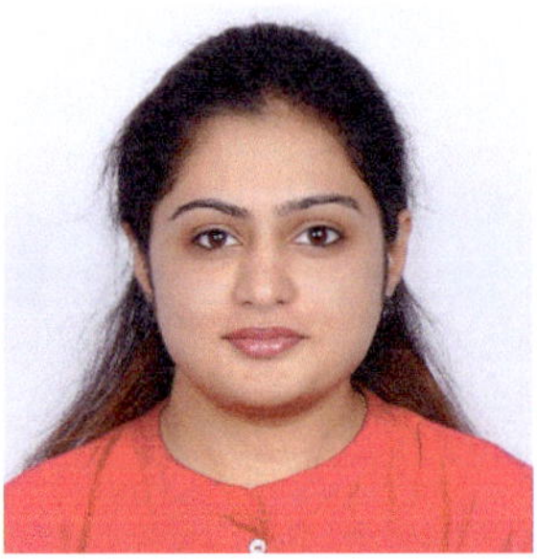

**Varsha Arer** is a PhD student in the Department of Biotechnology, Ramaiah University of Applied Sciences, Bangalore, and a lecturer at KLE Dental Sciences, Bangalore. She studies $\beta$-lactamases and their role in antimicrobial resistance mechanisms. Her work involves the identification of potential drug targets and the exploration of their interactions, aiming to contribute valuable insights to the field.

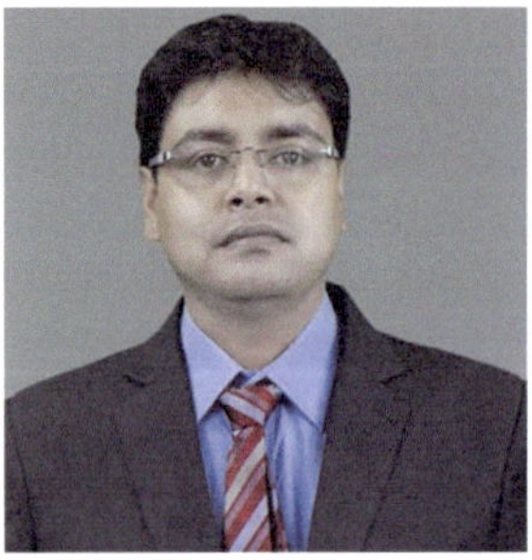

**Dr. Debasish Kar** completed his PhD at the Department of Biotechnology, IIT Kharagpur. He is currently an assistant professor in the Department of Biotechnology, M.S. Ramaiah University of Applied Sciences. His research interests involve unraveling the mechanisms of antimicrobial resistance in Gram-negative bacteria.

# Illustrator

**Aaron Menezes** completed his bachelor's in St. Xavier's College, Mumbai, and is currently pursuing his master's at S.I.E.S College, Mumbai.

# The History of Antibiotics

# 1

Deepesh Nagarajan

**Abstract**

The timeline of antibiotic discovery can be divided into three ages: the dawn, the golden age, and the dark age. The dawn of antibiotic discovery involved the discovery of salvarsan, prontosil, and penicillin. The golden age followed in the 1960s during which all families of antibiotics in clinical use today were discovered. During the current dark age, very few antibiotics have been discovered, as the cost per new antibiotic developed has exponentially increased. This chapter will discuss all ages of antibiotic discovery, with an emphasis on the dark age and Eroom's law.

**Keywords**

Eroom's law · Drug discovery · Drug development

Antibiotics are chemical substances produced by various microorganisms, or made synthetically, that are capable of destroying (bactericidal) or inhibiting (bacteriostatic) the growth of other microorganisms.

D. Nagarajan (✉)
Department of Biotechnology, M.S. Ramaiah University of Applied Sciences, Bangalore, India

Department of Microbiology, St. Xavier's College, Mumbai, India
e-mail: deepeshn.bt.ls@msruas.ac.in; deepesh.nagarajan@xaviers.edu

© The Editor(s) (if applicable) and The Author(s), under exclusive license to Springer Nature Singapore Pte Ltd. 2024



D. Nagarajan (ed.), *Antibiotics and Their Mechanisms of Action*,
https://doi.org/10.1007/978-981-97-6851-6_1

## 1.1 The Dawn of an Era

The word "antibiotics," literally meaning *life-killing*, was first used by **Selman Waksman**, a Ukrainian-American soil microbiologist, who went on to discover over 20 different antibiotics [1]. He discovered **Streptomycin**, the first aminoglycoside in 1943, which was the first antibiotic treatment of tuberculosis.

In 1909, while **Paul Ehlrich** was working on the antibacterial effects of dyes, he discovered **salvarsan** (Fig. 1.1): an arsenic-based chemical, which proved to be useful in the treatment of syphilis. Although salvarsan can be considered the first truly antimicrobial agent, it could not technically be classified as an antibiotic as it was proven to be toxic to its patients [2].

Salvarsan's greatest contribution to medical science came in the form of **Prontosil**, discovered by **Josef Klarer** and **Fritz Mietzsch** in 1932 [3], carrying on Ehlrich's work. **Ernest Fourneau** and **Jacques Tréfouël** [4] demonstrated that Prontosil was a prodrug that was metabolized to sulfanilamide. This paved the way for the creation of an entire family of sulfa drugs.

The first antibiotic, **Penicillin**, was a serendipitous discovery made in 1928 by **Alexander Fleming** (Fig. 1.2). **Ernst Chain** and **Howard Florey** helped produce penicillin on an industrial scale, thereby playing an important role in turning this accident into a medical breakthrough [5].

It is interesting to note that the first clinically used drug was prepared by **Rudolph Emmerich** and **Oscar Löw** in 1899: **pyocyanase** from *Pseudomonas aeruginosa* [6] (Fig. 1.3). This treatment was eventually abandoned, since the results were inconsistent and the preparation process was extremely toxic.

## 1.2 The Golden Age

The discovery of the first three antimicrobials salvarsan, prontosil, and penicillin laid the foundations for modern medicine. The principles and processes developed during the discovery of these early antimicrobial agents paved the way for other researchers to discover and produce a large number of antibiotics.

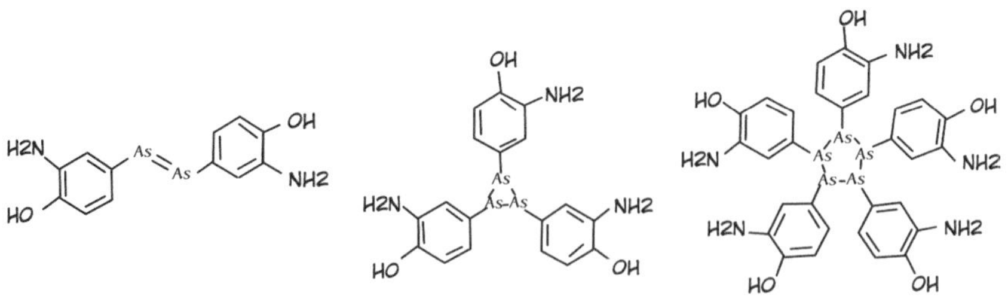


**Fig. 1.1** Salvarsan in solution can exist in a range of oligomerization states. Shown here (from left to right) are a dimer, a trimer, and a pentamer. Oligomerization occurs via the arsenic–arsenic covalent bonds

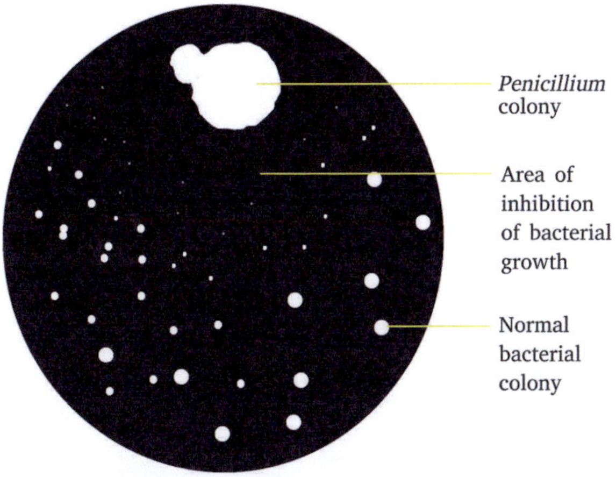


**Fig. 1.2** Alexander Fleming's original plate displaying inhibition of Staphylococci by a penicillium colony (artist's impression)

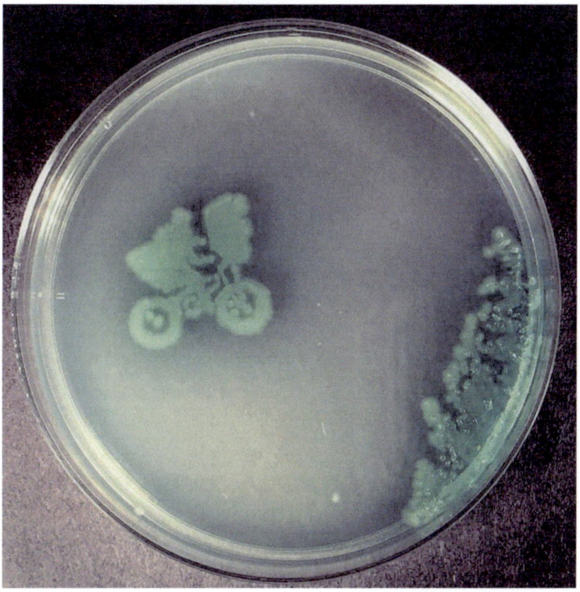

**Fig. 1.3** Petri art created using *Pseudomonas aeruginosa*. Pyocyanase was isolated from this organism (previously named *Bacillus pyocyaneus*). Image credit: Dr. Courtney Toth (University of Toronto, University of Calgary)

The golden age of antibiotic discovery in the 1950s and 1960s immediately followed (Fig. 1.4) [7]. Half of all antibiotics in use today, and all antibiotic families, were discovered in this period. Although most of these antibiotics are still in clinical use, their effectiveness has significantly decreased over time due to an inevitable increase in antibiotic resistance.

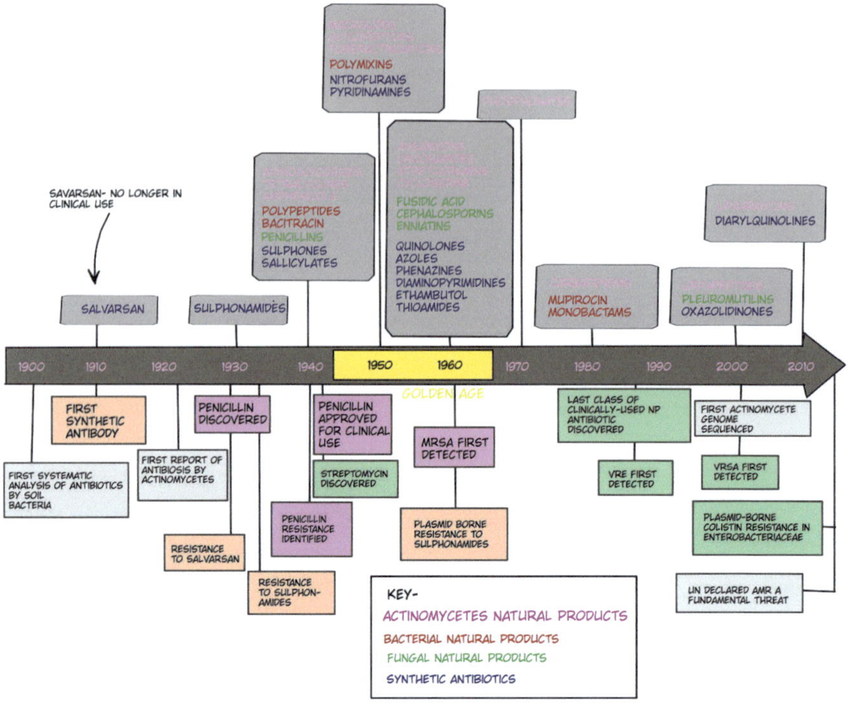


**Fig. 1.4** **Timeline of antibiotic development** and important events in antibiotic history. A disproportionate number of new antibiotics were discovered during the golden age. Antibiotics are colored according to the sources they were extracted from. MRSA = methicillin-resistant *Staphylococcus aureus*, VRE = vancomycin-resistant enterococci, VRSA = vancomycin-resistant *S. aureus*

## 1.3 The Dark Age and Eroom's Law

Following the golden age, there has been a steady decline in the rate of antibiotic discovery coupled with an increase in antimicrobial resistance. These two phenomena herald the dark age of antibiotic discovery. Eroom's law [8] can help establish the existence of this dark age:

> **Definition 1.1 Eroom's law**: The number of new drugs approved by the US Food and Drug Administration per billion USD spent (inflation adjusted) has **halved roughly every 9 years** (Fig. 1.5).

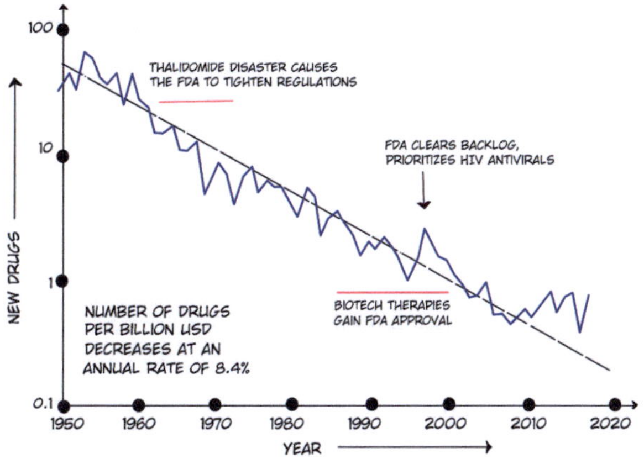


**Fig. 1.5** **Eroom's law**: the exponential decrease in the number of approved drugs with time

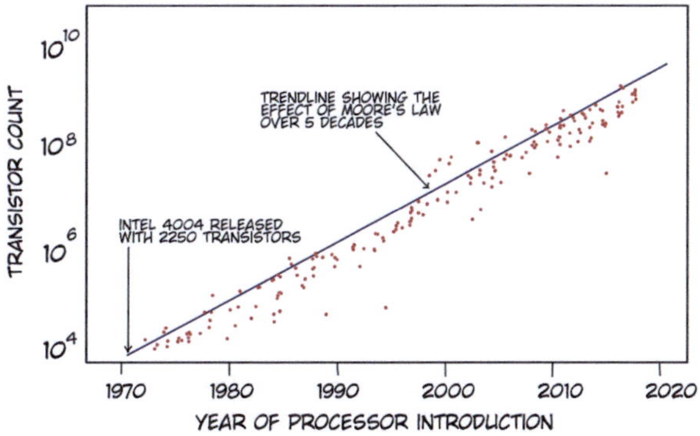


**Fig. 1.6** **Moore's law**: the exponential increase in the number of transistors per CPU with time

Contrast Eroom's law with Moore's law:

**Definition 1.2** **Moore's law**: The number of transistors in a dense integrated circuit (IC) **doubles every 2 years** (Fig. 1.6).

Moore's law tracks the continuing advancement of an important field. Eroom's law in contrast tracks the continued regression of an arguably even more important field. To understand the current state of drug discovery, one must understand the causes of Eroom's law:

### 1.3.1 Better Than the Beatles?

Imagine a world where every successive rock band was legally compelled to be superior to its predecessor. In such an environment, very little new music would be made. This idea serves as a useful analogy to understand the current state of drug regulation. New drugs will not be approved unless they are markedly superior to an existing approved drug. This means that drugs that could have been potential blockbusters (and approved) if released a few decades ago may now be considered inferior to generic drugs that treat the same illness (and therefore not approved).

As an example, a new class of anti-ulcerants (soraprazan, discontinued) could not compete with $H_2$ receptor antagonists and proton pump inhibitors despite being excellent drugs if evaluated in isolation.

### 1.3.2 The Cautious Regulator

Progressively lowering risk tolerance causes regulators to become more and more conservative and have very strict rules and regulations when approving new drugs. For example, the 1962 Kefauver Harris Amendment was passed following the Thalidomide tragedy and the ensuing birth defects, making drug companies legally obliged to report serious side effects.

### 1.3.3 Basic Research–Brute Force Bias

This is the tendency to overestimate the ability of high-throughput molecular biology methods and new brute force screening methods.

In the 1950s and 1960s drugs were simply identified based on their *in vitro* and *in vivo* efficacy (mouse models). Today, drug discovery (Fig. 1.7) begins at the "target": a protein molecule that, if inhibited, can kill a pathogen or disrupt a metabolic pathway. Molecules that bind to this target are called "hits." Hits are then verified and optimized to become "leads." A case study of a drug discovery project using this approach is provided in Infobox 1.3.4.

Technology exists today that allows for the screening of thousands of molecules against a target to check for binding: surface plasmon resonance, biolayer interferometry, nuclear magnetic resonance, or simply colorimetry combined with automated plate readers. This approach, however, is flawed because the underlying

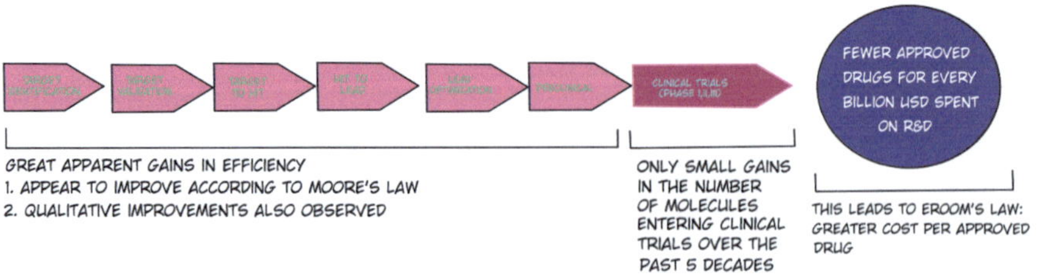


**Fig. 1.7 The drug discovery pipeline**: The probability that a new drug candidate completes clinical trials has remained constant over 50 years despite substantial apparent progress in the early stages of the pipeline. One explanation is that the community has simply optimized the "wrong" processes

assumption is that one drug binds to one target, whereas older drugs are now known to bind to several targets (off-target effects).

### 1.3.4 "Throw Money at It" Tendency

If it does not work, throw money at it: This is the tendency to add excessive human resources and other resources to research and development, leading to a huge rise in expenditure. This tendency may compound the other reasons for spiraling drug development costs but is not a causative agent by itself.

**Infobox 1.1**

**Open Source Drug Discovery: A Case Study**

Open Source Drug Discovery (OSDD) was a Council of Scientific and Industrial Research (CSIR) program launched in 2008 with ambitious goals of developing drugs against a variety of diseases prevalent in India, such as tuberculosis, HIV, and malaria [9]. The program was designed around the idea of decentralizing the process of drug discovery. Anyone with any level of education could contribute to drug discovery, using open source molecular docking software and, if needed, using hardware provided by the program. CSIR laboratories and other volunteers interested in the project were then expected to procure and experiment on the drugs developed computationally by volunteers.

The program was extremely ambitious in scope and received USD 12 million in initial funding from the Indian government. At its peak, the program boasted 7500 participants from all across the world who were involved in 110 research projects. The program also boasted some initial successes, including:

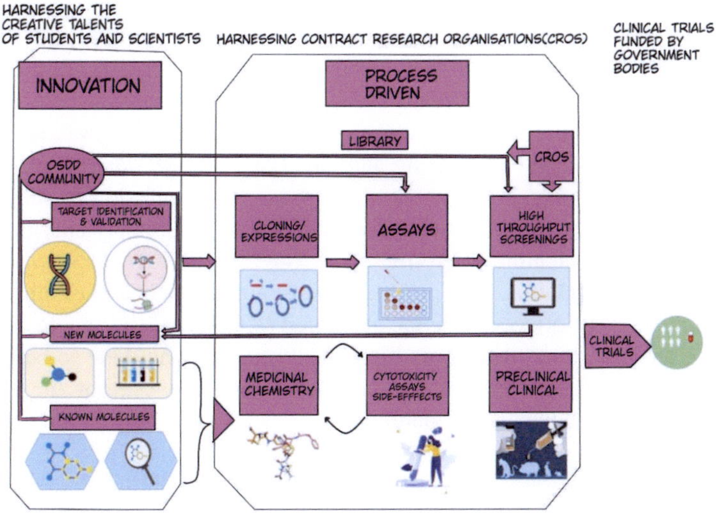

1. The sequencing and annotation of the *Mycobacterium tuberculosis* genome [10]
2. Computationally identifying 49 compounds as potential inhibitors of *M. tuberculosis* mycolyltransferase antigen 85 [11]
3. Improved tools for bioenergetic calculations [12] and toxicity prediction [13]

The Open Source Drug Discovery Consortium published ten papers in total. Despite these successes, the program fell far short of its initial goal: to develop drugs. **No drugs developed by the consortium were approved for clinical use**. No drugs developed by the consortium even entered clinical trials. The project was *de facto* canceled in 2014 when the Indian government did not allocate further funding for it [14].

What caused the failure of this program? In retrospect, it is easy to point out its many faults:

1. **Lack of resources.** The project was only allocated a few tens of millions of dollars over its entire run. Developing even a single drug can cost as much as a billion USD.
2. The program heavily relied on **computational methods for drug design**. Most computational drug design strategies follow the **"one target–one drug"** approach. Thousands to millions of drug candidates are virtually screened *in silico* against a crystal structure or computational model of a protein deemed to be essential for metabolism. The best binders are then screened *in vitro*. In hindsight, we know that designing a drug for a single target is an unproductive approach (see Sect. 1.3.3). Drugs, especially antibiotics, can have multiple off-target effects which all contribute to their efficacy. Unfortunately, the OSDD project was launched in 2008 before these ideas permeated through the field.
3. **Lack of trained personnel.** The project relied heavily on volunteers who were usually undergraduate students with little to no training in the field of bioinformatics. Chemoinformaticians, medicinal chemists, and clinicians were scarcely represented due to a shortage of such personnel in the country [15].
4. **Project mismanagement.** Initially the OSDD consortium was reluctant to publish its work on sequencing and annotating the *M. tuberculosis* genome in a peer-reviewed journal [16], thereby implicitly refusing to subject it to scrutiny by experts in the field. Such a decision is extremely unusual for any public sector scientific enterprise.
5. **Exaggerated claims.** The project's chief coordinator made unsubstantiated claims that the project made the annotated *M. tuberculosis* genome available "for the first time," despite multiple institutions having done so before [16]. Doing so eroded trust for the project in both the eyes of the scientific community and the general public.

## 1.4 Problems

**Problem 1.1**

What prerequisites needed to be met before the golden age of drug discovery occurred? Why did not the golden age occur in 1860, for example, right after Louis Pasteur proposed the germ theory of disease?

**Problem 1.2**

You are the CEO of a start-up biotech firm focusing on the development of new drug molecules. Your lead scientist has asked you for money for the following projects:

1. Expanding the animal house, containing mice, rats, and rabbits. He wishes to test more compounds *in vivo*.
2. A new computational cluster. He wants to test more drug molecules against a predetermined target *in silico*, which he believes will save precious laboratory time and materials.
3. Whole genome sequencer: to sequence the genomes of various pathogenic bacterial strains to try and identify new drug targets.
4. Expanded organic chemistry laboratory: to add a greater assortment of functional groups to your companies' existing drug molecules. It is hoped that doing so will broaden their spectrum of activity and improve their half-life in human blood.

You can only fund two projects. Which projects do you pick?

**Problem 1.3**

A counterargument against Eroom's law can be made: The cause of the decline in the number of new drugs approves is not due to the aforementioned problems, but because:

1. The pharmaceutical industry has become cartelized and formed a bureaucratic oligopoly, resulting in reduced innovation and efficiency. A total of 20 Big Pharma companies control the majority of global branded drug sales [17].
2. Big Pharma has reduced investment in research and development, spending double on marketing, and has focused on elevating drug prices instead of risk-taking.

Do you agree or disagree with this counterargument? Explain.

**Problem 1.4**

As a policymaker, what steps would you take to reverse the trend described by Eroom's law?

## References

1. The history of antibiotics. https://web.archive.org/web/20220107033752/https://microbiologysociety.org/members-outreach-resources/outreach-resources/antibiotics-unearthed/antibiotics-and-antibiotic-resistance/the-history-of-antibiotics.html. Accessed: 7 JAN 2022
2. Gould K (2016) Antibiotics: from prehistory to the present day. J Antimicrobial Chemotherapy 71(3):572–575
3. Brownlee G (1949) The sulphonamides and allied compounds. Nature 163(4148):662–662
4. Trefouel J, Nitti F, Bovet D (1935) Activité du p-aminophénylsulfonamide sur les infections streptococciques expérimentales de la souris et du lapin. CR Soc de biol (Paris) 120:756–758
5. Discovery and development of penicillin. https://web.archive.org/web/20220201044755/https://www.acs.org/content/acs/en/education/whatischemistry/landmarks/flemingpenicillin.html. Accessed: 1 FEB 2022
6. Aminov RI (2010) A brief history of the antibiotic era: lessons learned and challenges for the future. Front Microbiol 1:134
7. Hutchings MI, Truman AW, Wilkinson B (2019) Antibiotics: past, present and future. Current Opinion Microbiol 51:72–80
8. Scannell JW, Blanckley A, Boldon H, Warrington B (2012) Diagnosing the decline in pharmaceutical r&d efficiency. Nature Rev Drug Discovery 11(3):191–200
9. Singh S (2008) India takes an open source approach to drug discovery. Cell 133(2):201–203
10. Bhardwaj A, Bhartiya D, Kumar N, Scaria V, Open Source Drug Discovery Consortium, et al. (2009) TBrowse: an integrative genomics map of Mycobacterium tuberculosis. Tuberculosis 89(5):386–387
11. Gahoi S, Mandal RS, Ivanisenko N, Shrivastava P, Jain S, Singh AK, Raghunandanan MV, Kanchan S, Taneja B, Mandal C, et al. (2013) Computational screening for new inhibitors of M. tuberculosis mycolyltransferases antigen 85 group of proteins as potential drug targets. J Biomol Struct Dynam 31(1):30–43
12. Kumari R, Kumar R, Open Source Drug Discovery Consortium, Lynn A (2017) g_mmpbsa a GROMACS tool for high-throughput MM-PBSA calculations. J Chem Inf Model 54(7):1951–1962
13. Gupta S, Kapoor P, Chaudhary K, Gautam A, Kumar R, Open Source Drug Discovery Consortium, Raghava GPS (2013) In silico approach for predicting toxicity of peptides and proteins. PLoS One 8(9):e73957
14. Nagarajan R (2014) Funds dry up for drug discovery project
15. Pulla P (2014) The collateral benefits of India's open source drug discovery programme
16. Jayaraman KS (2010) India's tuberculosis genome project under fire. Nature News 9
17. Danzon PM (2014) Competition and antitrust issues in the pharmaceutical industry. CRC America Latina-Centro Regional de Competencia para America Latina

# Methods of Antibiotic Discovery

# 2

Deepesh Nagarajan

**Abstract**

Antibiotic discovery has relied on a diverse variety of methods: traditional culturing methods, which involve the creation of zones of inhibition on solid media, chemical modification of natural antibiotics, and high-throughput screening, involving the automates testing of thousands of molecules to find "hits" or "leads." Newer methods and concepts such as computer-aided drug design and drug rediscovery are also discussed.

**Keywords**

Culture methods · iChip · ADME · Lipinski's rules · High-throughput screening · CADD · Drug rediscovery

The development of new antibiotics remains a crucial tool in the fight against drug-resistant pathogens. Methods of antibiotic discovery vary from simple cultural methods used to discover antibiotics during the golden age to modern computational design approaches which while advanced still have to prove their worth.

D. Nagarajan (✉)
Department of Biotechnology, M.S. Ramaiah University of Applied Sciences, Bangalore, India

Department of Microbiology, St. Xavier's College, Mumbai, India
e-mail: deepeshn.bt.ls@msruas.ac.in; deepesh.nagarajan@xaviers.edu

© The Editor(s) (if applicable) and The Author(s), under exclusive license to Springer Nature Singapore Pte Ltd. 2024

D. Nagarajan (ed.), *Antibiotics and Their Mechanisms of Action*,
https://doi.org/10.1007/978-981-97-6851-6_2

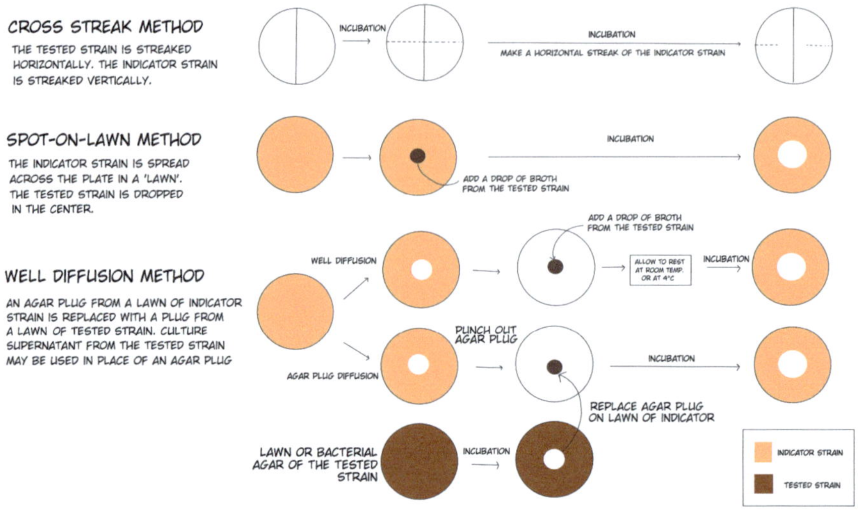


**Fig. 2.1** **Solid culture methods**: the cross-streak, spot-on-lawn, and well diffusion methods [1]

## 2.1 Culture-Based Approaches

In the 1940s, the soil microbiologist Selman Walksman screened soil bacteria for antagonisms, and his approach is still used today. The culture methods are based on one common principle, that is, of inhibiting a test strain over a closely cultivated indicator strain. It is presumed that the test strain will produce an antimicrobial compound which will target the indicator strain [1]. A variety of techniques can be used to detect antimicrobial activity in solid cultures, such as the cross-streak method, the spot-on-the-lawn method, and the well diffusion method (Fig. 2.1). We will now briefly look at each of these methods.

### 2.1.1 The Cross-Streak Method

This technique is simple and effective for screening, but the test and indicator strains are required to have the same conditions of temperature, atmosphere, and growth duration. The test strain is vertically inoculated on an agar plate. The incubation time is determined by the moment secondary metabolites are excreted. The indicator strain is then horizontally inoculated, and the plate is reincubated. A line of inhibition is expected in the indicator strain.

### 2.1.2 The Spot-on-Lawn Method

This method involves a lawn of indicator strain, on which a drop of test strain is deposited. It is then incubated after which a zone of inhibition is expected around the drop of test strain.

### 2.1.3 The Well Diffusion Method

The principle behind the well diffusion method is that the diffusion of antimicrobials through agar inhibits susceptible species. An agar plate is pooled with indicator strain, and agar holes are bunched out aseptically, forming wells. There are two main variants of this method:

1. **Agar plug diffusion**: A cylinder of agar is removed from a plate inoculated with the test strain which is placed into the well of the indicator plate.
2. A **liquid broth** of the test strain is placed in the well of the indicator plate.

In both the spot-on-lawn and well diffusion methods, the expected zone of inhibition is observed after an optimal rest time at 4 °C.

### 2.1.4 iChip: Cultivating the "Uncultivable"

Only a small fraction of microbial species can be artificially cultivated, making a majority of the microbiological population uncultivable [2]. The field of drug discovery has therefore only explored a tiny fraction of available microbial biodiversity. It is entirely conceivable that entirely new classes of antibiotics could be isolated from uncultivable organisms. Approaches to cultivate such organisms are therefore urgently required.

Soil (or any other natural environment) contains an innumerable number of **undiscovered growth factors** absent in standard laboratory media; factors that are essential to the growth of uncultivable organisms. One approach to supplying uncultivable organisms with these growth factors involves **shifting laboratory cultivation into the environment**. The ichip follows this approach [3, 4] and is specifically designed for culturing unculturable soil bacterium.

The components of the ichip are illustrated in Fig. 2.2.

The ichip was used to isolate several antibiotic candidates including teixobactin [5], a peptide-like secondary metabolite capable of inhibiting cell wall synthesis in *Staphylococcus aureus* and *Mycobacterium tuberculosis*.

Despite these successes, the ichip suffers from the following drawbacks:

1. The ichip cannot culture organisms that need to be in close proximity to a synergetic partner.

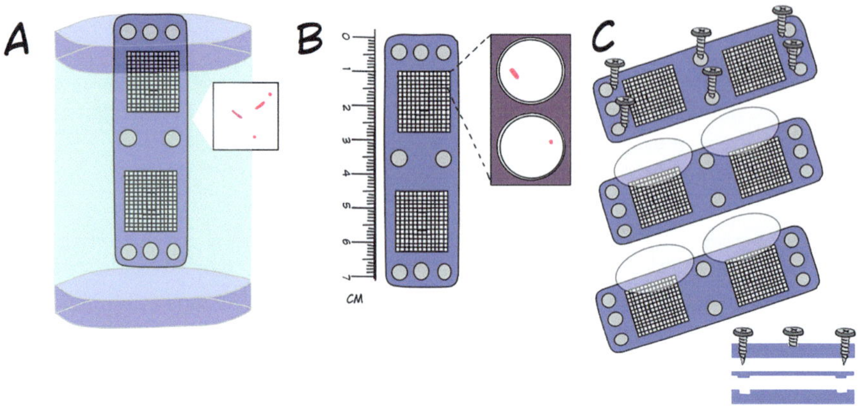


**Fig. 2.2** **Conceptual schematics of the ichip** [2]: **(a)** A **central plate** is designed containing multiple "through-holes." This plate is dipped into a bacterial suspension. **(b)** The bacterial solution containing potentially uncultivable organisms must be diluted such that **each through-hole on average captures one bacterium**. **(c)** Assembly of the device: The through-holes are covered by membranes on either side. These membranes allow for the diffusion of small molecules. Matching holes on the upper and lower plates align with holes on the central plate. Once pressure-sealed, the (upper plate)-(membrane)-(central plate)-(membrane)-(lower plate) assembly acts like an **isolated diffusion cell**. The ichip must then be placed in the organisms' native environment (usually soil) to allow growth factors into the diffusion cell

2. A considerable amount of moisture is required in the environment in order to prevent drying up of the gelling agent present inside the ichip.
3. Placing the ichip on the surface of aquatic sediments leads to an anoxic condition which creates an unnatural environment for the cells in the ichip.

## 2.2 Chemical Modification

Natural antibiotics are chemically modified through the addition of functional groups to the parent structure. These functional groups may either be small methyl, hydroxyl, amide, or chloro groups or may even include long functionalized aliphatic side chains. Chemical modification of existing antibiotics is an **empirical rather than rational** process: The effect of a chemical modification is usually unknown until the desired molecule is synthesized and experimentally tested.

Rational approaches to chemical modification of antibiotics also exist, the most recognized being **Lipinski's rules of 5**. These rules were formulated in 1997 by Christopher A. Lipinski and can be used to distinguish between drug-like and nondrug -like molecules. Drug-like molecules are expected to possess satisfactory ADME properties (Infobox 2.2). The rules are as follows:

1. No more than **5 hydrogen bond donors**
2. No more than **10 hydrogen bond acceptors**

3. A molecular mass ≤**500 Dalton**
4. An **octanol–water partition coefficient** (log P) that is ≤ 5

Lipinski's rules are merely "rules of thumb." They are not based on any actual biophysical constraints. Only about 50% of orally administered new chemical entities actually obey them.

Almost all antibiotic families have been developed via chemical modification of a parent natural antibiotic. This includes the **penicillin** (Sect. 3.2), **quinolone** (Sect. 6.2), and **tetracycline** (Sect. 8.2) families. A parent structure is chemically modified to improve solubility, increase spectrum of activity, improve pharmacokinetic properties, and overcome resistance to the parent compound.

► **Remark**

**Rationalism** is the belief that all knowledge can be derived from reason and logic alone. In contrast, **empiricism** is the belief that all knowledge must be derived from experience and experimentation within the physical world. Despite originating in the field of philosophy, these two schools of thought are mirrored in different approaches to drug discovery.

**Infobox 2.1**

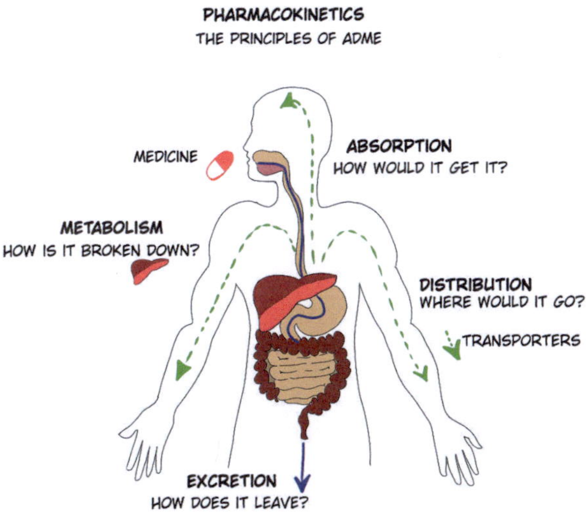


Pharmacokinetics involves studying a drug's journey through the body. This journey can be broken down into four different stages: absorption, distribution, metabolism, and excretion (ADME).

1. **Absorption** deals with the drugs' immediate journey from its point of administration (oral, intramuscular, intravenous, and subcutaneous).

2. **Distribution** describes the journey of the drug through the body, usually through the bloodstream. Distribution begins where absorption ends. Distribution ends when the drug reaches its site of action. For antibiotics, this site of action is usually an infected tissue or organ.
3. **Metabolism** deals with biochemical processes that break down the drug. Such processes usually occur in the liver and bloodstream.
4. **Excretion** deals with the elimination of the drug from the body. Drugs can be excreted via urine, feces, sweat, saliva, tears, bile, and breast milk.

An ideal drug possesses ideal ADME properties. It should be easily administered and readily absorbed. It should reach the site of action rapidly and in sufficient concentrations. It should possess a high serum half-life. It should not damage the liver or other organs during metabolism. It should not damage the kidneys or other organs during excretion. Chemical modification techniques attempt to improve a drug's ADME properties to reach these ideals.

## 2.3 High-Throughput Screening

For every million screened compounds, only one marketable drug emerges (Fig. 2.3). Therefore the drug industry is incentivized to screen ever larger libraries of drugs. High-throughput screening (HTS) is a drug discovery process that involves screening a large number of chemical and/or biological compounds against specific biological target at rates exceeding a thousand per day. The goal of HTS is to identify molecules that bind to the target and inhibit its activity.

Biological targets are usually proteins deemed to participate in essential metabolic processes, without which the pathogen cannot survive. Examples include the bacterial 70S ribosome (see Chap. 8), DNA gyrase (see Chap. 6), RNA polymerase (see Chap. 7), and dihydrofolate reductase (see Chap. 11). Such proteins are extracted and purified for use in high-throughput, automated assays. Simple colorimetric/enzymatic assays can be performed in great volumes on 96-, 192-, 384-, 1536-, 3456-, or 6144-well plates by automated devices. Alternate assays include high-throughput circular dichroism, surface plasmon resonance (SPR), and nuclear magnetic resonance (NMR) that probe for structural changes within the target to confirm binding to a compound.

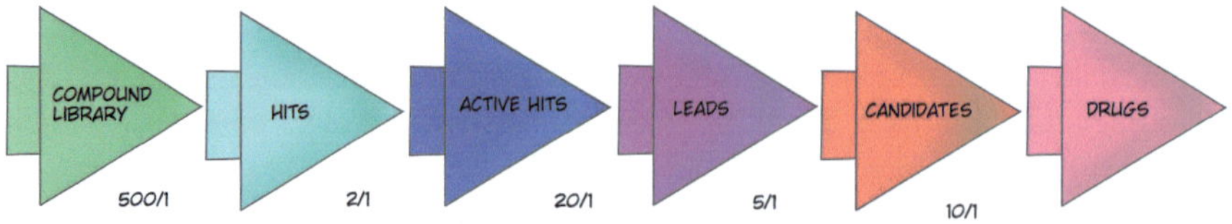


**Fig. 2.3** High attrition at every stage of the drug discovery pipeline

Compounds that bind and inhibit a target of interest are called **hits** or **leads**. After the hits have been successfully identified, the drug-likeness of the compound needs to be predicted. Hits may then be optimized with respect to toxicity, potency, selectivity, and pharmacokinetics in an *in vitro* environment before they can be moved forward along the drug discovery pipeline.

Despite the apparent advantages, HTS has failed to dramatically increase the number of antibiotics approved for clinical use. This is because:

1. The **one drug–one target** axiom upon which HTS is based is not necessarily correct (see Sect. 1.3.3). An antibiotic may need to interact with several unknown targets to be fully effective. This is something HTS cannot capture accurately. Testing antibiotics on whole cells rather than single molecules may therefore be a more productive approach.
2. Large numbers of **false positives** can be generated. The *in vivo* efficacy of a compound that inhibits an isolated target *in vitro* is by no means guaranteed.

## 2.4 Computer-Aided Drug Design

▶ **Remark**

Know your Latin:
***In cerebro***: A thought experiment, performed in one's mind
***In silico***: An experiment performed in silicon, therefore on a computer
***In vitro***: An experiment performed outside an organism, traditionally using glassware
***In vivo***: An experiment performed inside an organism

Computer-aided drug design (CADD, Fig. 2.4) is a branch of drug design that uses various chemical–molecular and quantum methods to discover, design, and develop new drugs.

The main role of CADD is to computationally filter and select compounds for *in vitro* tests. Virtual screening helps find *in silico* hits for a target of interest. Computational screens require far less time and resources than experimentally testing every single compound, even if a high-throughput screen is used. Therefore an extraordinarily large number of compounds (regularly ranging in the millions) can be assessed using CADD. CADD can also be used for lead optimization.

CADD has made significant development toward treating illnesses such as influenza, AIDS, glaucoma, and non-small-cell lung cancer [6]. Most notably, CADD approaches have contributed to the discovery and design of HIV-1 integrase inhibitors [7].

Different CADD approaches can be classified into three broad categories:

1. **Structure-based methods**: These methods require the 3D, all-atom structure of the target. 3D structures of the target and ligand are docked together and

**Fig. 2.4 The CADD pipeline**: steps usually taken during *in silico* screening

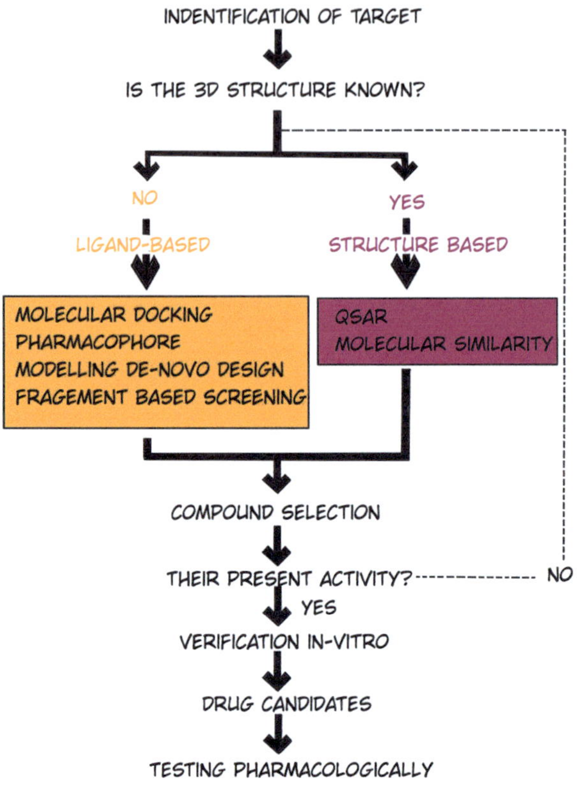


scored using an energy function. Best-scoring ligands may then be tested *in vitro*. Structure-based methods are also used for the interpretation of the mechanism of action of active molecules at the molecular level, thermodynamic assessment of the ligand-target recognition, and depiction of binding sites, e.g., molecular docking and molecular dynamics.

2. **Ligand-based methods**: These methods focus on the chemical structure and biological activity of ligands and are typically used for lead optimization: to enhance the activity of existing active molecules. Alternatively, they may be used when the structure of the target is unknown, e.g., similarity searching and QSAR (quantitative structure–activity relationship) modeling.
3. **Hybrid and end point-based methods**: These methods involve a combination of structure-based and ligand-based methods, e.g., some approaches to pharmacophore modeling.

The field of CADD has great potential, and despite rapid progress in recent years it has still not yet reached maturity. Our understanding of biochemistry and biomolecular forces is limited; therefore biomolecular interactions can only be modeled with low accuracy. The most CADD predictions are wrong.

## 2.5 Drug Rediscovery

Due to the paucity of new drugs developed during the current dark age of antibiotic discovery and due to the increasing threat of drug resistance, there has been an elevated interest in "rediscovering" old antibiotics and putting them to use [8]. Older antibiotics withdrawn from clinical use may once again be used to treat pathogens that have developed resistance against newer antibiotics. Alternatively, old antibiotics may be repurposed to treat different emerging diseases.

All old antibiotics are FDA approved. Their pharmacokinetic properties, toxicity, and side effects are extensively documented in the literature. Rediscovering an old drug is therefore far more cost-effective than developing a new drug.

Some examples of rediscovered drugs are as follows:

1. **Doxycycline**:

   - **Traditionally useful against**: traveler's diarrhea, Rocky Mountain spotted fever, sinusitis, syphilis, trachoma, balantidiasis, brucellosis, chancroid, and plague
   - **New uses**: Lyme disease, pneumonia, animal bites, STDs, chlamydia infections, and ehrlichiosis

2. **Minocycline**:

   - **Traditionally useful against**: anthrax, cholera, gonorrhea, leptospirosis, severe acne, trachoma, and yaws
   - **New uses**: central nervous system (CNS) infection with susceptible organisms, CNS Lyme disease Legionnaires' disease, and methicillin-resistant *S. aureus* (MRSA) infections

3. **Trimethoprim/sulfamethoxazole**:

   - **Traditionally useful against**: chancroid, chronic bronchitis, chronic granulomatous disease, Citrobacter infections, acute sinusitis, Aeromonas infections, traveler's diarrhea, and urinary tract infections.
   - **New uses**: Nocardia infections, Legionella infections, Listeria infections, and meningitis

4. **Metronidazole**:

   - **Traditionally useful against**: *Entamoeba histolytica* infections, hepatic Amebiasis, intra-abdominal infections, and pelvic infections
   - **New uses**: Antibiotic-associated colitis, antibiotic-associated diarrhea, and *Clostridium difficile* infections

▶ **Remark**

**Drug repurposing** is another approach to discovering drugs that is closely related to drug rediscovery. While rediscovery involves using an existing antibiotic to treat different bacterial infections, repurposing involves using an existing drug of any nature to treat a disease of any etiology. An example of drug repurposing involves using **Sildenafil**, initially approved for treating angina (chest pain), for treating erectile dysfunction.

## 2.6 Problems

**Problem 2.1**

Your guide hands you an organism that he isolated from the Methi riverbank. He believes it secretes a compound capable of inhibiting the growth of six strains of carbapenem-resistant *Pseudomonas spps* that his pathologist collaborator sent him. Design a simple experiment to confirm.

**Problem 2.2**

You have confirmed that the organism in Problem 2.1 inhibits *Pseudomonas spps*. Unfortunately, your organism becomes nonviable after 5–10 passages in LB media. You only have a finite supply of lyophilized stock culture. Suggest a method to culture this organism indefinitely.

**Problem 2.3**

Compare and contrast high-throughput screening with computer-aided drug design. Are *in silico* or *in vitro* techniques more reliable? Name an antibiotic discovery technique with a proven track record that is superior to both methods.

**Problem 2.4**

Does Ampicillin obey Lipinsky's rule of five?
Does tigecycline obey Lipinsky's rule of five?
Explain for both.

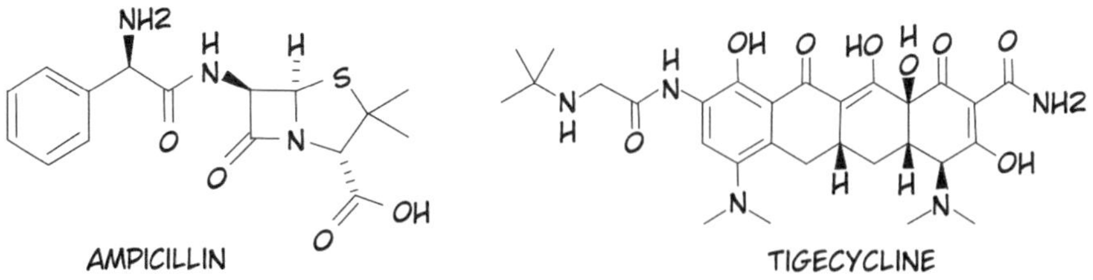

## References

1. Durand GA, Raoult D, Dubourg G (2019) Antibiotic discovery: history, methods and perspectives. Int J Antimicrobial Agents 53(4):371–382
2. Nichols D, Cahoon N, Trakhtenberg EM, Pham L, Mehta A, Belanger A, Kanigan T, Lewis K, Epstein SS (2010) Use of ichip for high-throughput in situ cultivation of "uncultivable" microbial species. Appl Environ Microbiol 76(8):2445–2450
3. Kaeberlein T, Lewis K, Epstein SS (2002) Isolating "uncultivable" microorganisms in pure culture in a simulated natural environment. Science 296(5570):1127–1129
4. Berdy B, Spoering AL, Ling LL, Epstein SS (2017) In situ cultivation of previously uncultivable microorganisms using the ichip. Nature Protocols 12(10):2232–2242
5. Ling LL, Schneider T, Peoples AJ, Spoering AL, Engels I, Conlon BP, Mueller A, Schäberle TF, Hughes DE, Epstein S, et al. (2015) A new antibiotic kills pathogens without detectable resistance. Nature 517(7535):455–459
6. Prieto-Martínez FD, López-López E, Juárez-Mercado KE, Medina-Franco JL (2019) Computational drug design methods—current and future perspectives. In silico drug design, pp 19–44
7. Liao C, Nicklaus MC (2010) Computer tools in the discovery of hiv-1 integrase inhibitors. Future Med Chem 2(7):1123–1140
8. Cunha BA (1997) New uses for older antibiotics: The 'rediscovery' of four beneficial and cost-effective antimicrobials. Postgraduate Med 101(4):68–88

# 3 Penicillin

Deepesh Nagarajan

**Abstract**

Penicillin is a $\beta$-lactam antibiotic discovered by Alexander Fleming. Today, a range of natural and synthetic $\beta$-lactam drugs have entered the clinic. Penicillin's mechanism of action involves the inhibition of cell wall synthesis by binding to transpeptidase: the enzyme that forms tetrapeptide linkages in the peptidoglycan component of the cell wall. The mechanism of action of penicillin can be deciphered from simple experiments with protoplasts lacking a cell wall. Delving deeper, penicillin's observed substrate analogy with (D-ala)-(D-ala) leads to the discovery of transpeptidases. Penicillin binding to transpeptidase can be confirmed by a range of experiments, including affinity chromatography, the SYPRO Orange thermal shift assay, and X-ray crystallography. Bacteria evolve resistance to penicillin via mutations to transpeptidase, the evolution of $\beta$-lactamases, and the use of multidrug efflux pumps.

**Keywords**

Penicillin · $\beta$-lactam · ESBL · $\beta$-lactamase · Antibiotic resistance

Penicillins are a group of antibiotics discovered and obtained from the mold *Penicillium chrysogenum* (formerly *Penicillium notatum*). The penicillins were the first in their class of **$\beta$-lactam** antibiotics (Fig. 3.1), of which there are 60+ examples in clinical use at the time of writing.

D. Nagarajan (✉)
Department of Biotechnology, M.S. Ramaiah University of Applied Sciences, Bangalore, India

Department of Microbiology, St. Xavier's College, Mumbai, India
e-mail: deepeshn.bt.ls@msruas.ac.in; deepesh.nagarajan@xaviers.edu

© The Editor(s) (if applicable) and The Author(s), under exclusive license to Springer Nature Singapore Pte Ltd. 2024



D. Nagarajan (ed.), *Antibiotics and Their Mechanisms of Action*,
https://doi.org/10.1007/978-981-97-6851-6_3

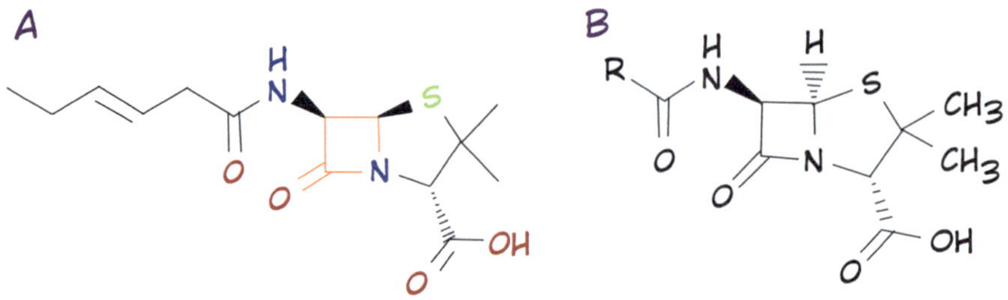


**Fig. 3.1** **(a) Structure of Penicillin F**: the first penicillin variant purified by Howard Florey and Ernst Chain in 1940. The $\beta$-lactam ring is highlighted in orange. **(b) Penicillin core structure**. "R" is a variable group. Different penicillin derivatives will have different chemical moieties in place of "R"

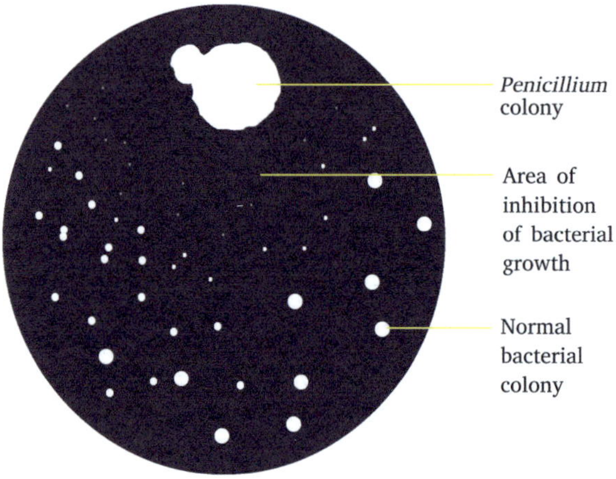


**Fig. 3.2** Alexander Fleming's original plate displaying inhibition of Staphylococci by a penicillium colony (artist's impression)

## 3.1 History

Penicillin was serendipitously discovered by **Alexander Fleming** in 1928, after he noticed mold growing on a petri dish meant to culture Staphylococci (Fig. 3.2) [1]. This mold exerted a zone of inhibition on all bacterial colonies attempting to grow near it, indicating that it was producing an antimicrobial compound.

Although Fleming discovered penicillin, he was never able to produce it on an industrial scale. **Howard Florey** and **Ernst Chain** discovered how to isolate and concentrate the antibiotic (Penicillin F), using it in a clinical trial for the first time in 1941. Florey went on to mass-produce the antibiotic for American wartime requirements during World War II (Fig. 3.3). All three men won the 1945 Nobel Prize in Physiology or Medicine.

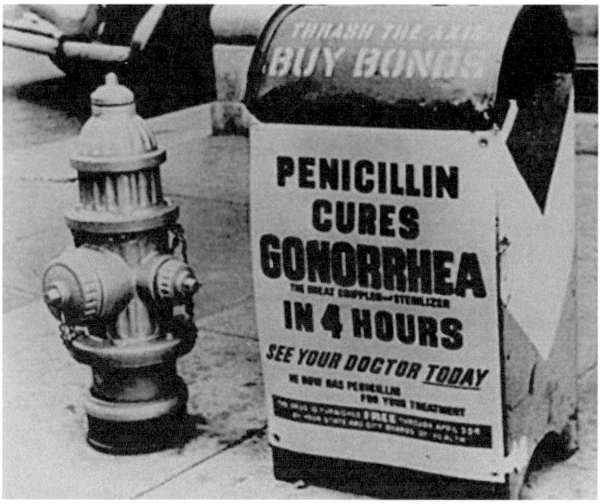


**Fig. 3.3** Penicillin advertisement for World War 2 American servicemen, circa 1944

## 3.2 Classes of Penicillins

A full list of all penicillin drugs and the classes they belong to is provided in Table 3.1.

### 3.2.1 Natural Penicillins

**Penicillin G** was the first mass-produced antibiotic, lending the "-cillin" name to all penicillin derivatives that followed. Although revolutionary for the time, it could not be consumed orally and had to be injected into patients. **Penicillin V** was therefore created as a modified variant that was stable in stomach acid and could be consumed orally. Both are narrow-spectrum drugs that were effective against gram-positive streptococci and a few gram-negative organisms like meningococci and *Treponema pallidum*. Despite their historic contributions, widespread drug resistance has made both Penicillin G and V nearly obsolete for clinical use.

### 3.2.2 Aminopenicillins

Aminopenicillins have a relatively broad spectrum of activity. **Ampicillin** can be used both orally (acid stable) and parenterally, whereas **amoxicillin** is used primarily orally. These drugs are $\beta$-lactamase sensitive. Amoxicillin is also part of triple therapy used to treat *Helicobacter pylori* infections, alongside clarithromycin and a proton pump inhibitor to reduce stomach acids.

**Table 3.1** Penicillin derivatives and their classes

| Natural penicillins | Spectrum |
|---|---|
| Penicillin G/benzylpenicillin | Narrow |
| Penicillin V | Narrow |
| **Aminopenicillins** | |
| Ampicillin | Broad |
| Amoxicillin | Broad |
| **Penicillinase-resistant penicillins (Antistaphylococcal penicillins)** | |
| Methicillin | Narrow |
| Oxacillin | Narrow |
| Cloxacillin | Narrow |
| Dicloxacillin | Narrow |
| Nafcillin | Narrow |
| Flucloxacillin | Narrow |
| **Extended Spectrum Penicillins (Antipseudomonal Penicillins)** | |
| Azlocillin | Broad |
| Carbenicillin | Broad |
| Mezlocillin | Broad |
| Piperacillin | Broad |
| Ticarcillin | Broad |
| **$\beta$-lactamase inhibitors** | |
| Clavulanic acid | |
| Tazobactam | |

### 3.2.3 Penicillinase-Resistant Penicillins

**Methicillin** was initially used as a second-line drug to deal with resistant organisms, as it is insensitive to $\beta$-lactamases (bacterial enzymes that break open the $\beta$-lactam ring). However, the emergence of MRSA (methicillin resistant *Staphylococcus aureus*) has seen **oxacillin** replacing methicillin in this role. **Nafcillin**, **cloxacillin**, **dicloxacillin**, and **flucloxacillin** are other related antibiotics.

### 3.2.4 Extended Spectrum Penicillins

**Piperacillin/tazobactam**, **Azlocillin**, **Carbenicillin**, **Mezlocillin**, and **Ticarcillin** are particularly useful for combating *Pseudomonas aeruginosa*. **Tazobactam** is a heavily modified penicillin that serves as a $\beta$-lactamase inhibitor. **Mezlocillin** is excreted by the liver, and therefore it is useful for biliary tract infections, such as cholangitis (inflammation of the bile duct). **Ticarcillin** is also one of the few antibiotics capable of treating infections caused by *Stenotrophomonas maltophilia*.

## 3.3 Mechanism of Action

**Penicillin inhibits cell wall synthesis**. It does this by inhibiting the transpeptidase enzyme that catalyzes the final step in cell wall biosynthesis, the cross-linking of peptidoglycan (Fig. 3.4).

The best way to understand penicillin's mechanism of action is to retrace and understand the original experiments performed for its elucidation. The subsections below will guide you through every step of the process:

### 3.3.1 Inhibition of Cell Wall Synthesis

Despite being discovered in 1928, there was no consensus in the scientific community about its mechanism of action until as late as 1956 as described in a note [2] published by Joshua Lederberg at the time (Fig. 3.5).

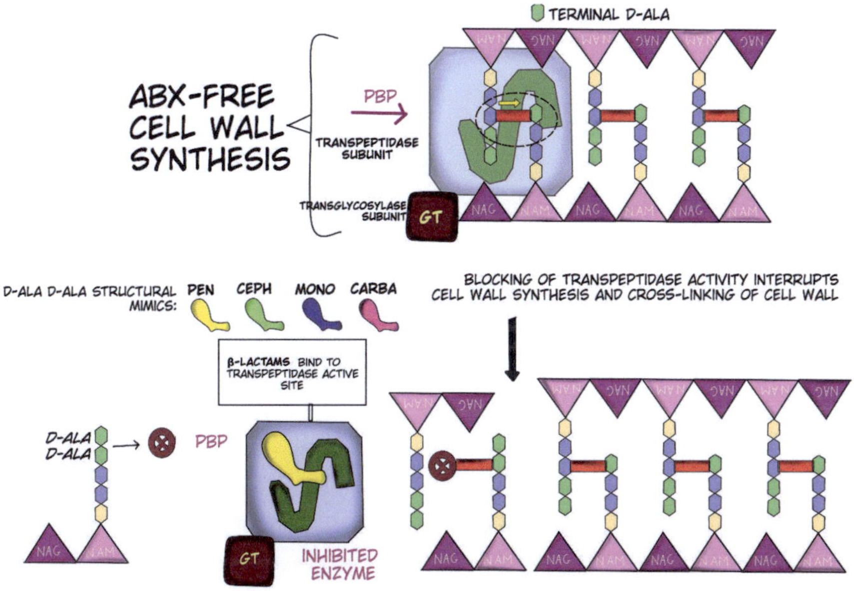


**Fig. 3.4** **Penicillin's molecular mechanism of action**: Transpeptidase is an enzyme that binds to the terminal (D-ala)-(D-ala) residues catalyzing the covalent linkage (cross-linking) of peptides from different peptidoglycan chains and expelling one D-ala in the process. Penicillin binds to the transpeptidase active site, blocking its activity and interrupting cell wall cross-linking

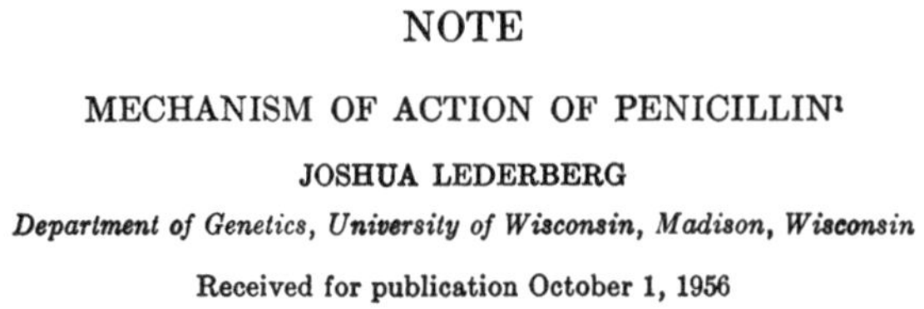

NOTE

MECHANISM OF ACTION OF PENICILLIN[1]

JOSHUA LEDERBERG

*Department of Genetics, University of Wisconsin, Madison, Wisconsin*

Received for publication October 1, 1956

**Fig. 3.5** Joshua Lederberg very succinctly described early experiments to determine penicillin's mechanism of action in his 1956 one-page note to the Journal of Bacteriology. You are strongly encouraged to read it [2]. He would win the 1958 Nobel Prize in Physiology or Medicine for unrelated reasons

The first step toward understanding penicillin's mode of action was through the development **protoplasts**. Using the K-12 strain of *Escherichia coli*, it was observed that:

1. Incubating *E. coli* with penicillin for 2 hours caused it to form a "protoplast." A protoplast is a large, spherical, osmotically fragile cell.

> **Inference 3.1** The cell wall maintains bacterial shape. *E. coli* is typically rod-shaped. If an *E. coli* protoplast loses its shape in the presence of penicillin, then penicillin must be targeting the cell wall.

2. Protoplasts cannot survive in normal media. They will balloon and lyse if not maintained in hypertonic media containing a high concentration of sucrose and $MgSO_4$.

> **Inference 3.2** After penicillin causes pathogens to lose their cell walls, they die due to osmotic fragility. They can no longer survive in isotonic body fluids.

3. If these same protoplasts are incubated in hypertonic media but in the absence of penicillin, they regain their original morphology.
4. These reformed *E. coli* are viable and can be incubated in normal isotonic media.

These observations are illustrated in Fig. 3.6.

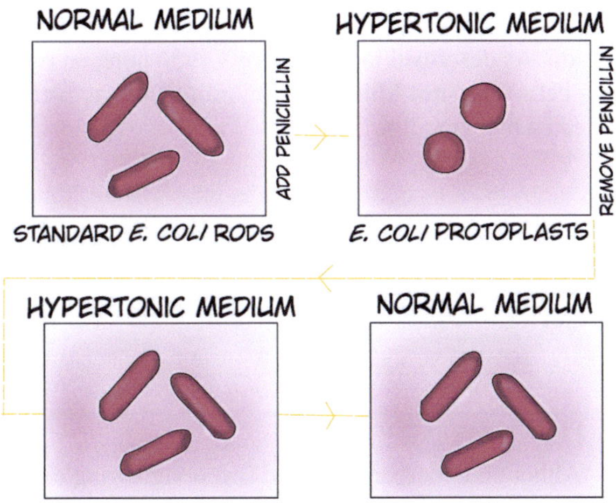


**Fig. 3.6** Formation of *E. coli* protoplasts and the return of the original *E. coli* morphology (artist's Impression)

*E. coli* protoplasts are formed in the presence of penicillin. *E. coli* protoplasts regain their original morphology in the absence of penicillin. It is therefore fair to conclude that **penicillin is responsible for the loss of bacterial cell walls**.

## Proposed experiment 3.1

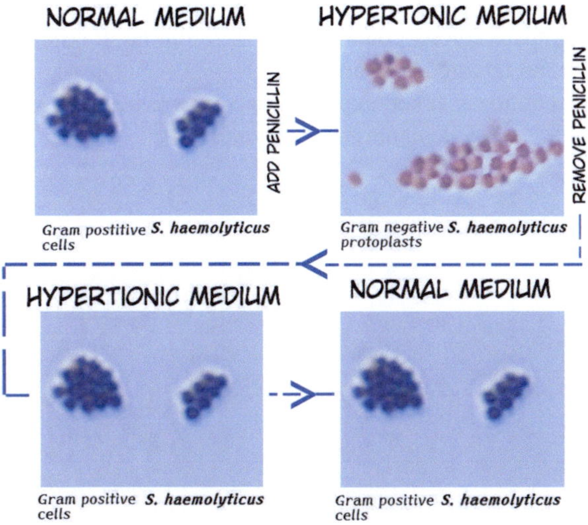


Another experiment can be performed to more directly observe the penicillin-induced loss of the bacterial cell wall.

Rather than using *E. coli*, protoplasts can be formed from a gram-positive organism like *Staphylococcus haemolyticus*. Using *S. haemolyticus* allows one to directly **observe the loss of the bacterial cell wall using Gram staining**.

Other early experiments also helped shed light upon penicillin's mechanism of action. As described in Lederberg's 1956 note, an experiment found that **nongrowing cells were not killed** by penicillin. Only actively dividing cells appeared to be affected by penicillin.

**Inference 3.3** If only active cells are targeted by penicillin, then penicillin does not target the existing cell wall. Instead, **penicillin must be targeting new cell wall formation.**

**Proposed experiment 3.2**

Although Lederberg claimed that nongrowing cells were not killed by penicillin, he never described or cited an experiment to verify this claim in his 1956 note. Thankfully, it is very easy to design such an experiment.

The easiest way to obtain nongrowing cells is to force them into the stationary phase. This can be accomplished by growing bacteria (*E. coli*) in nutrient broth initially, then pelleting down the culture, and resuspending it in saline. Physiological saline (0.85% NaCl) offers no nutrients. Incubation in saline for 48 hours should be sufficient to induce dormancy in bacteria.

Once stationary, perform a colony count (A). Incubate dormant *E. coli* in penicillin for 2 hours. Dilute out the penicillin, and perform another colony count (B). Compare colony counts A and B. If similar, it confirms that dormant organisms are not targeted by penicillin.

There are countless other experimental approaches you can use to verify Lederberg's claim. Try designing one by yourself!

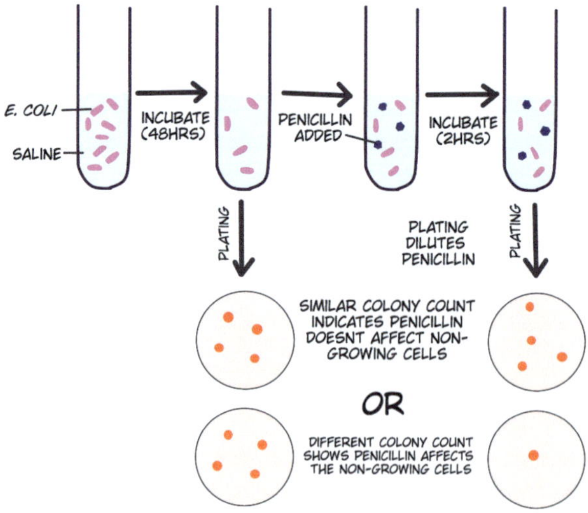

### 3.3.2 Inhibition of Transpeptidases

**Technique 3.1**

Two affinity chromatographic techniques are used to isolate transpeptidases:

**Covalent affinity chromatography**. This technique uses penicillin itself (or any other ligand of interest) to bind to transacetylases. This technique is no longer preferred because penicillin has to be covalently linked to its substrate and because the column will purify all penicillin binding proteins.

**NiNTA affinity chromatography**. Currently the preferred choice for purifying proteins out of crude extracts. NiNTA-labeled agarose beads are commercially available and do not have to be custom-made. HIS-tags, composed of six sequential histidines, are only present on the artificially tagged protein and nowhere else. HIS-tags are typically added to the ends of the protein gene inserted into the plasmid.

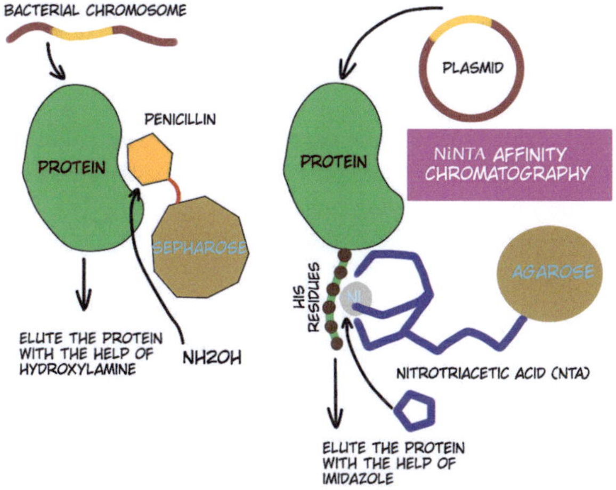


In 1965, it was noted that one of the conformations of penicillin matched one of the conformations of D-ala-D-ala, part of the peptidoglycan precursor [3] (Fig. 3.7). This hints at penicillin being a **substrate analog**.

At the time transpeptidase enzymes were not discovered. However, the existence of the tetrapeptide linkage implied the existence of an enzyme to create it. Likewise, the existence of penicillin implied that this hypothetical enzyme bound to (D-ala)-(D-ala).

The first transpeptidase was reported in 1966 [4]. It was studied in a crude cell-free extract of *E. coli*. Since then, hundreds of transpeptidase sequences have been discovered. Early purification methods used penicillin (covalent) affinity chromatography to isolate natural transpeptidases from bacterial lysates [5]. Today nickel-NTA purification columns are preferred.

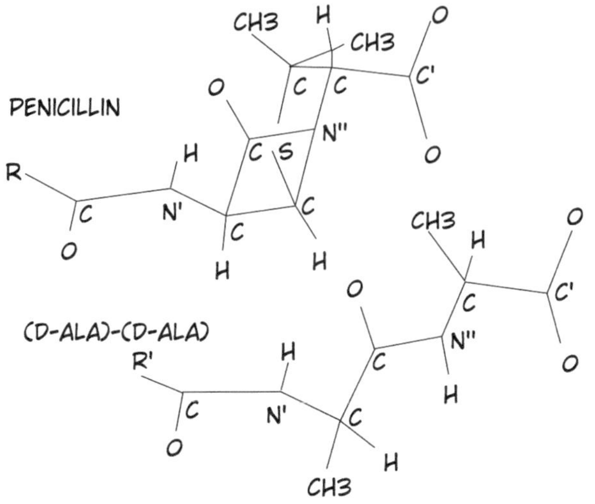


**Fig. 3.7** The structures of two conformations of penicillin and (D-ala)-(D-ala) placed side to side for comparison

The first experiments to determine penicillin binding on isolated transpeptidase (or carboxypeptidase, a closely related enzyme) were performed using complicated and expensive experiments involving radiolabeled penicillin [6]. Such experiments have largely been superseded by far simpler biophysical assays, such as the SYPRO Orange thermal shift assay.

SYPRO Orange is typically not only used to understand protein folding and stability, but it can also be used to study protein–ligand interactions.

Proteins that bind to ligands (like penicillin) are far more stable in their bound form than in their unbound form. Therefore, transpeptidases bound to penicillin can resist thermal denaturation far better than unbound transpeptidases when assayed using SYPRO Orange (Fig. 3.8) [7].

The ultimate confirmation of binding comes from structural data. Ideally, X-ray crystallographic or nuclear magnetic resonance (NMR) data should show the protein bound to the ligand and at the expected ligand binding site.

One example of a structural study on a transpeptidase comes from a report on its X-ray crystal structure solved in complex with carbenicillin, a penicillin derivative [7] (Fig. 3.9). Note that this is the same study that reported the SYPRO Orange binding data.

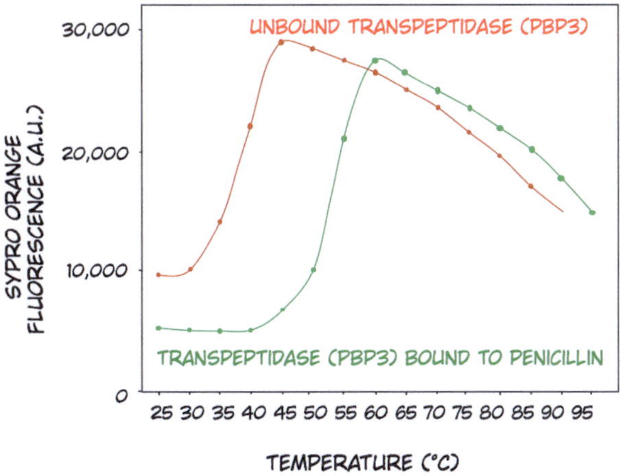


**Fig. 3.8** SYPRO Orange used to confirm carbenicillin (penicillin derivative) binding for transpeptidase/penicillin binding protein 3 (PBP3) from *P. aeruginosa* [7]

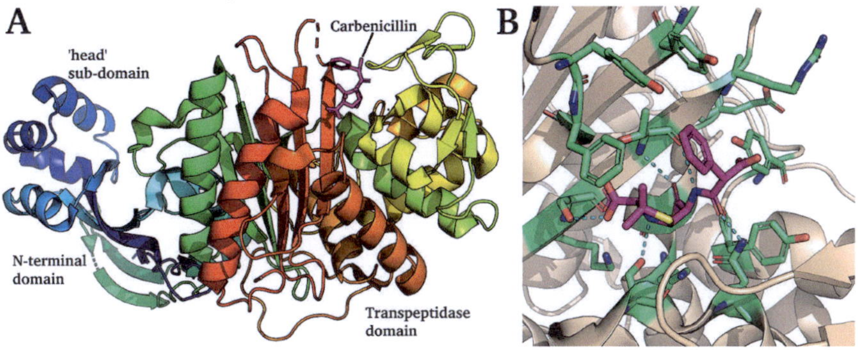


**Fig. 3.9** X-ray structure of **carbenicillin** (penicillin derivative) **in complex with transpeptidase**/penicillin binding protein 3 (PBP3) from *P. aeruginosa*. PDB ID: 3ocl [7]. **(a)** The entire protein structure consisting of two domains is shown. A domain is a large, independently folding substructure within a single protein chain. **(b)** A close-in of carbenicillin (magenta) along with all of the protein residues that interact with it. Hydrogen bonds are shown as cyan dotted lines. Oxygen atoms (hydrogen bond acceptors) are colored red. Nitrogen atoms (hydrogen bond donors) are colored blue

**Technique 3.2**

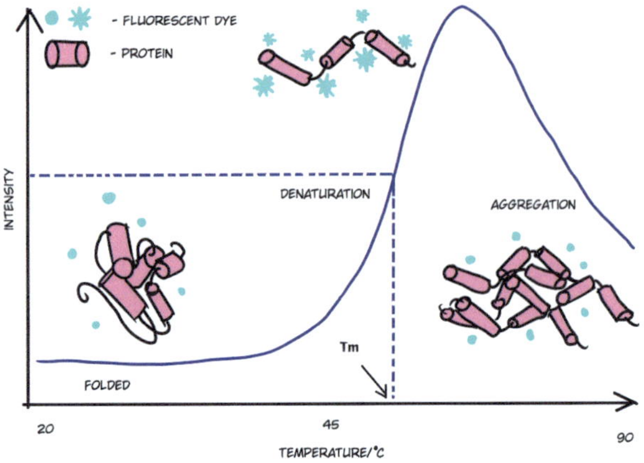


The **SYPRO Orange thermal shift assay**. Proteins contain hydrophobic cores and hydrophilic exteriors. When heat is used to denature proteins, the protein chain unfolds and exposes its hydrophobic residues to aqueous solvent.

SYPRO Orange is a hydrophobic fluorescent dye. It will preferentially bind to exposed hydrophobic residues on protein chains. Furthermore, SYPRO Orange will only fluoresce when it is bound to these exposed hydrophobic residues. Therefore, fluorescence can be used to track protein unfolding with increasing temperature.

A well-folded protein typically has only low baseline fluorescence. Fluorescence increases as temperature increases, culminating in a peak. Beyond the peak, unfolded protein begins to aggregate, shielding hydrophobic residues from solvent and decreasing fluorescence.

**Proposed experiment 3.3**

**Laboratory evolution of resistance** coupled with **gene sequencing** can verify transpeptidase activity of putative transpeptidases without having to isolate or characterize the enzymes *in vitro*.

Transform a penicillin-sensitive *E. coli* strain with a plasmid containing a penicillin-sensitive copy of any transpeptidase gene. Perform serial passages of this strain in media containing gradually greater concentrations of penicillin. Perform several replicates (10–20). Sequence all plasmids once resistance has evolved.

If your protein is a transpeptidase, then in at least some (but not necessarily all) of the replicates, you can expect to observe:

1. A number of mutations per gene much higher than the baseline rate. The baseline rate can be established by sequencing a noncoding insert into the plasmid or a genomic exon.

**Table 3.2** Mutations to transpeptidases/penicillin binding proteins (PBPs) of*Streptococcus gordonii*, showing the relationship between MIC, mutants per transpeptidase, and the total number of mutated transpeptidases [8]

| | | Mutation(s) in indicated gene | | | | |
|---|---|---|---|---|---|---|
| Isolate | MIC µg/mL | pbp1A | pbp1B | pbp2A | pbp2B | pbp2X |
| Parent | 0.008 | – | – | – | – | – |
| Mutants | | | | | | |
| PR1_0.25 | 0.25 | – | – | – | – | – |
| PR1_1 | 1 | – | – | – | – | $Q_{548}E$ |
| PR1_2 | 2 | – | – | – | – | $G_{545}S$ |
| | | | | | | $Q_{548}E$ |
| PR1_2ev | 2 | $H_{510}Y$ | – | – | $T_{450}A$ | $G_{545}S$ |
| | | | | | $V_{596}F$ | $Q_{548}E$ |

2. Strains possessing a higher MIC against penicillin should also possess a greater number of mutations in the transpeptidase gene than strains possessing a lower MIC.
3. Transforming a resistant plasmid into a sensitive strain of *E. coli* should confer penicillin resistance upon it.

Table 3.2 depicts the results of a laboratory evolution experiment for transpeptidases/penicillin binding proteins against penicillin [8]. Note how the number of mutants increases with MIC. Also note that the goal of this particular experiment was not to confirm transpeptidase activity of putative transpeptidases. However, the experimental techniques would be identical.

## 3.4 Penicillin Resistance Mechanisms

In his Nobel lecture in 1945, Fleming presciently warned about the dangers of misusing penicillin: *"It is not difficult to make microbes resistant to penicillin in the laboratory by exposing them to concentrations not sufficient to kill them, and the same thing has occasionally happened in the body."*

Just as Fleming had predicted, pathogens have developed a number of penicillin resistance mechanisms (Fig. 3.10). These range from ways to expel penicillin from the cytoplasm to cleaving the penicillin molecule altogether.

### 3.4.1 Transpeptidase Mutants

Mutations in the penicillin binding site in transpeptidase enzymes are a logical penicillin resistance mechanism (Table 3.2). A penicillin-resistant transpeptidase confers a four- to eightfold additional increase in penicillin resistance and is an

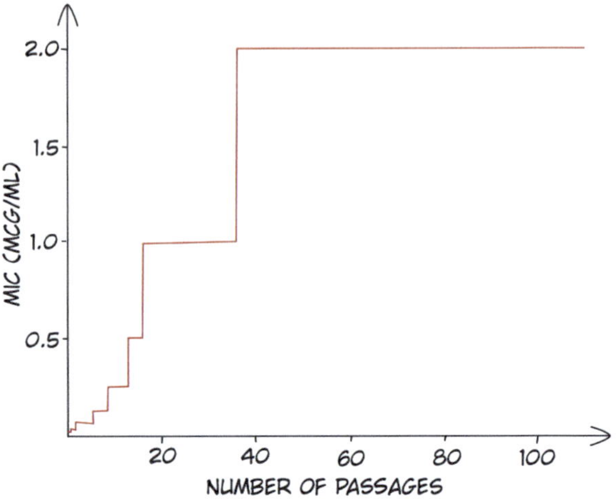


**Fig. 3.10** It is almost trivial to evolve penicillin resistance in a laboratory setting. Serial passages (subcultures) of an organism in media containing gradually increasing concentrations of penicillin can produce resistant mutants in as little as 1 month. The example here depicts the development of penicillin resistance in *Streptococcus gordonii* [8]

important first step in the development of penicillin resistance. However, higher MICs against penicillin can only be achieved through other resistance mechanisms.

Methicillin-resistant Staphylococci synthesize an additional penicillin binding protein (PBP) named PBP2a which has a much lower affinity for $\beta$-lactams than normal PBPs and is therefore capable of cell wall synthesis when the other $\beta$-lactams are inhibited.

Penicillin-resistant transpeptidases will display some common trends:

1. Strains possessing a higher MIC against penicillin should also possess a greater number of mutations in the transpeptidase gene, specifically within the (D-ala)-(D-ala)/penicillin binding site, than strains possessing a lower MIC.
2. All pathogens possess multiple transpeptidases. Therefore, strains possessing a higher MIC against penicillin should also possess a greater number of mutated transpeptidases.

### 3.4.2 $\beta$-Lactamases

$\beta$-Lactamases are enzymes that hydrolytically cleave (Fig. 3.11) the $\beta$-lactam ring of the penicillin molecule. $\beta$-lactamases can be classified into three subtypes depending on the backbone molecule cleaved (Fig. 3.12):

1. **Penicillinase** shows specificity for penicillin and its derivatives by hydrolyzing the $\beta$-lactam ring.
2. **Extended spectrum $\beta$-lactamases** (ESBLs) act against cephalosporin antibiotics.
3. **Carbapenemases** act against carbapenem antibiotics.

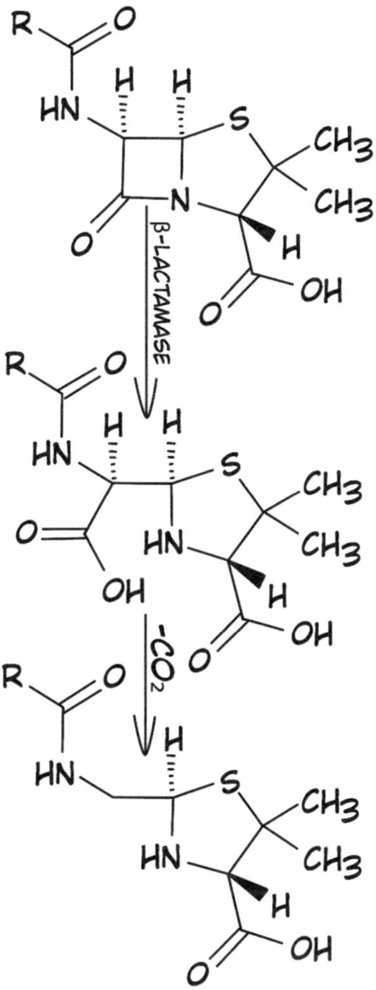


**Fig. 3.11** The $\beta$-lactamase reaction mechanism: The $\beta$-lactam ring is hydrolyzed creating an unstable carboxyl intermediate. This intermediate state loses $CO_2$, leaving behind a molecule with no antimicrobial properties

$\beta$-lactamases can be countered by $\beta$-lactamase inhibitors, which are coadministered with a $\beta$-lactam drug. $\beta$-lactamase inhibitors work by one of the two primary mechanisms:

1. They may become **substrates** that bind the $\beta$-lactamase enzyme with high affinity but form sterically unfavorable interactions. Examples include avibactam and relebactam.
2. They may also become **suicide inhibitors**, which permanently inactivate the enzyme through secondary chemical reactions in the active site. Examples include sulbactam, tazobactam, and clavulanic acid. Ampicillin–sulbactam, piperacillin/tazobactam (Zosyn), and amoxicillin/clavulanic acid (augmentin) are frequently used antibiotic/$\beta$-lactamase inhibitor combinations.

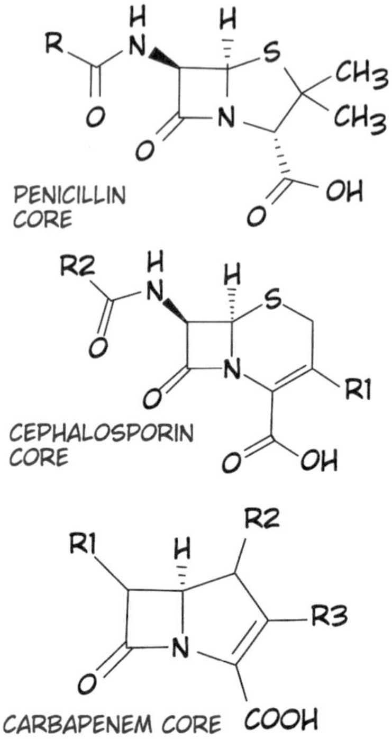


**Fig. 3.12** Core structures of penicillin, cephalosporins, and carbapenems, all of which contain the $\beta$-lactam ring. $\beta$-lactamases have evolved to hydrolyze $\beta$-lactam groups in almost every antibiotic

It should be noted that $\beta$-lactamases resistant to $\beta$-lactamase inhibitors have also been reported.

### 3.4.3 Multidrug Efflux Pumps

Multidrug efflux pumps are large, inner membrane proteins capable of recognizing several classes of antibiotics. Functionally, they "pump" drug molecules from the cytoplasm out into the periplasmic space or cell exterior while consuming ATP. Multidrug efflux pumps evolved to protect bacterial cells against small molecules and rogue amphiphilic compounds capable of crossing the plasma membrane. As such, they are also capable of expelling heavy metals, organic pollutants, plant-produced compounds, quorum sensing signals, and bacterial metabolites from the cytoplasm. Today they have been evolutionarily repurposed to target antibiotics which also need to be amphiphilic both to remain stable in aqueous solvents like serum and to be able to cross the plasma membrane.

At least a dozen multidrug efflux pump families have been documented [9] (such as the ABC transporters) (Fig. 3.13), each with their own mechanisms of action that are currently contested. However, there exists a general consensus that efflux pumps may act through three mechanisms:

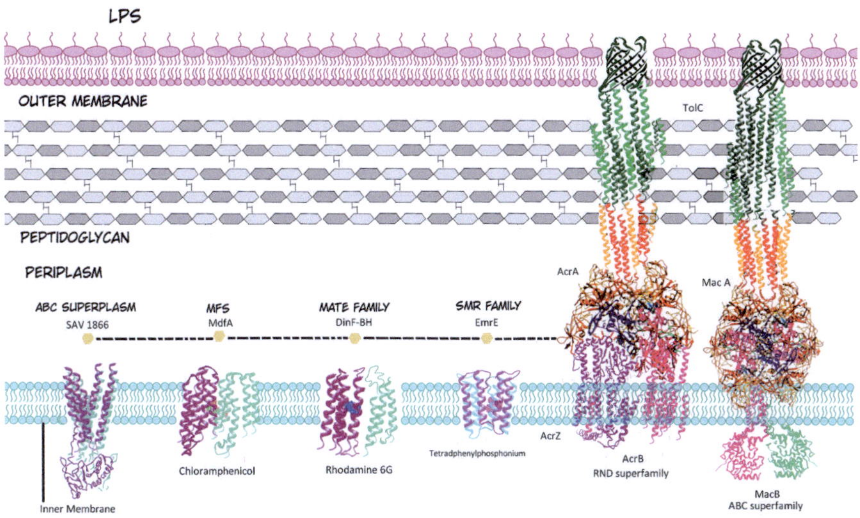


**Fig. 3.13** A sample of the structural diversity of known bacterial multidrug efflux pumps

1. **The classical pump**: Drug molecules in the aqueous phase at the cytosolic side of the plasma membrane interact with efflux pumps and are pumped across the membrane and released into the aqueous phase on the extracellular side.
2. **Vacuum cleaner model**: Hydrophobic drugs partition into the lipid bilayer and subsequently interact with efflux pumps, which then expel them into the aqueous phase on the extracellular side.
3. **Flippase model**: Drugs partition into the lipid bilayer, interact with a domain of efflux pumps within the cytoplasmic membrane leaflet, and are then translocated, or flipped, into the outer leaflet.

Multidrug efflux pumps have adapted themselves to expel almost every small drug molecule from the cytoplasm and are therefore counted as a mechanism of resistance for almost every cytosolic drug and not just penicillin.

## 3.5 Problems

### Problem 3.1

Your advisor hands you a protein gene on a plasmid. He suspects that the protein at hand is a transpeptidase. Unfortunately, the protein is extremely unstable and cannot be isolated *in vitro*. It is only stable in the cytoplasm and periplasmic space.

Design an experiment to determine whether the protein is a transpeptidase.

**Problem 3.2**

Your advisor hands you an experimental antibiotic with the following traits:

1. When incubates with *S. aureus* in a hypertonic medium, it induces the formation of protoplasts. Their formation was confirmed with a Gram stain.
2. Lyses *S. aureus* when in a stationary phase culture (after 48 h incubation in saline), confirmed with a colony count.

Your advisor then tells you that he is narrowed down the target of this drug to two possible molecules:

1. Peptidoglycan glycosyltransferase
2. N-acetylmuramic acid (NAM)

Which molecule is the more probable target? Why?

**Problem 3.3**

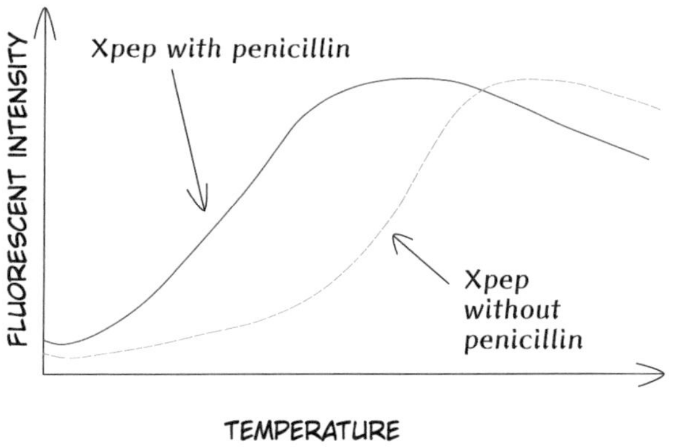


A project assistant has performed a SYPRO Orange thermal shift assay to determine whether a suspected transpeptidase (Xpep) binds to penicillin. Their results are attached alongside.
The project assistant insists that their data confirms penicillin binding to Xpep. Are they right or wrong? Why?

**Problem 3.4**

You have isolated a gene encoding a protein that is involved in penicillin resistance. You have inserted it into a plasmid and added a 6x HIS-tag at the C-terminal. You have narrowed down its mechanism of action to two possibilities:

1. A penicillin binding protein: It would act like a suicide substrate that binds to penicillin instead of transpeptidase.
2. A $\beta$-lactamase

Design an experiment to determine this protein's mechanism of action.

## References

1. Discovery and development of penicillin. https://web.archive.org/web/20220201044755/https://www.acs.org/content/acs/en/education/whatischemistry/landmarks/flemingpenicillin.html. Accessed: 1 FEB 2022
2. Lederberg J (1957) Mechanism of action of penicillin. J Bacteriol 73(1):144–144
3. Tipper DJ, Strominger JL (1965) Mechanism of action of penicillins: a proposal based on their structural similarity to acyl-D-alanyl-D-alanine. Proc Natl Acad Sci 54(4):1133–1141
4. Izaki K, Matsuhashi M, Strominger JL (1966) Glycopeptide transpeptidase and d-alanine carboxypeptidase: penicillin-sensitive enzymatic reactions. Proc Natl Acad Sci 55(3):656–663
5. Blumberg PM, Strominger JL (1972) Isolation by covalent affinity chromatography of the penicillin-binding components from membranes of *Bacillus subtilis*. Proc Natl Acad Sci 69(12):3751–3755
6. Yocum RR, Rasmussen JR, Strominger JL (1980) The mechanism of action of penicillin. penicillin acylates the active site of *Bacillus stearothermophilus* d-alanine carboxypeptidase. J Biol Chem 255(9):3977–3986
7. Sainsbury S, Bird L, Rao V, Shepherd SM, Stuart DI, Hunter WN, Owens RJ, Ren J (2011) Crystal structures of penicillin-binding protein 3 from *Pseudomonas aeruginosa*: comparison of native and antibiotic-bound forms. J Mol Biol, 405(1):173–184
8. Haenni M, Moreillon P (2006) Mutations in penicillin-binding protein (PBP) genes and in non-PBP genes during selection of penicillin-resistant *Streptococcus gordonii*. Antimicrobial Agents Chemotherapy 50(12):4053–4061
9. Du D, Wang-Kan X, Neuberger A, Van Veen HW, Pos KM, Piddock LJV, Luisi BF (2018) Multidrug efflux pumps: structure, function and regulation. Nature Rev Microbiol 16(9):523–539

# Vancomycin

# 4

Deepesh Nagarajan

**Abstract**

Vancomycin is a glycopeptide antibiotic discovered by Mack McCormick in 1955. Vancomycin is a transpeptidase analog. It binds to the terminal (D-ala)-(D-ala) residues on the peptidoglycan tetrapeptide, thereby preventing transpeptidase from binding and forming the tetrapeptide linkage. Vancomycin can be spectrophotometrically detected on the cell wall in a cell wall extract after sonication. More directly, BODIPY-tagged vancomycin can be visualized bound to the cell wall using phase contrast/fluorescent microscopy. *In vitro*, the binding of vancomycin to (D-ala)-(D-ala) can be confirmed by fluorometric titration against dansylated (D-ala)-(D-ala). X-ray crystallography can also be used to visualize the (D-ala)-(D-ala)-vancomycin complex. Vancomycin resistance evolves through D-ala → D-lac substitutions in the cell wall tetrapeptide.

**Keywords**

Vancomycin · Dansylation · Fluorescence microscopy · Antibiotic resistance

Vancomycin (Fig. 4.1) is a **glycopeptide** antibiotic used to treat a number of **gram-positive**, drug-resistant, and life-threatening infections such as *Staphylococcus aureus*, *Enterococcus spp.*, and *Clostridium difficile*. It is obtained from the soil bacterium *Amycolatopsis orientalis* and was discovered in 1955 by **Mack McCormick** working at Eli Lilly.

D. Nagarajan (✉)
Department of Biotechnology, M.S. Ramaiah University of Applied Sciences, Bangalore, India

Department of Microbiology, St. Xavier's College, Mumbai, India
e-mail: deepeshn.bt.ls@msruas.ac.in; deepesh.nagarajan@xaviers.edu

© The Editor(s) (if applicable) and The Author(s), under exclusive license to Springer Nature Singapore Pte Ltd. 2024

D. Nagarajan (ed.), *Antibiotics and Their Mechanisms of Action*,
https://doi.org/10.1007/978-981-97-6851-6_4

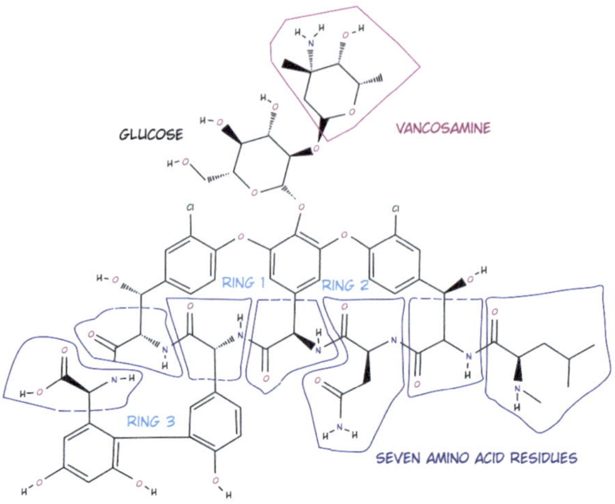


**Fig. 4.1** The structure of vancomycin showing the seven-membered nonribosomally synthesized peptide and the vancosamine-glucose disaccharide. The tricyclic ring system is created through both the standard peptide bond and through covalent linkages between noncanonical amino acid side chains

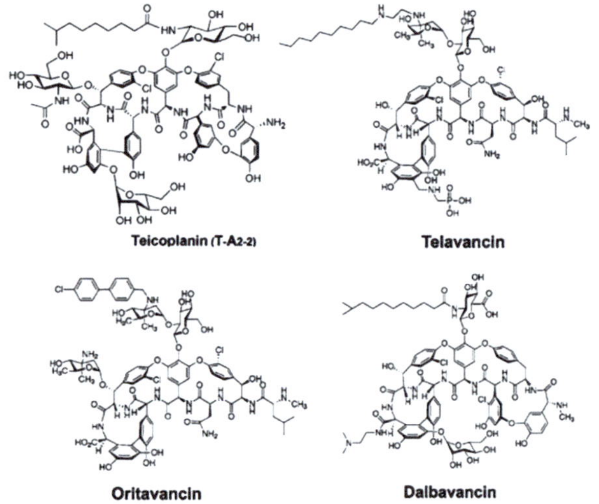


**Fig. 4.2** Other members of the glycopeptide family. The structures of **Teicoplanin**, **Oritavancin**, **Telavancin**, and **Dalbavancin** are shown

Structurally, vancomycin is highly complex. It consists of a seven-membered peptide chain forming a tricyclic ring system. This ring system has a disaccharide composed of vancosamine and glucose attached to it. Due to this complexity, its structure was only determined in 1981.

Vancomycin is biosynthesized via a complex system of nonribosomal protein synthesis. The total chemical synthesis of vancomycin independent of any biological systems was a long-standing goal of chemists and has only recently been accomplished.

Despite its efficacy, vancomycin and other glycopeptides (Fig. 4.2) are considered to be drugs of last resort due to their adverse side effects that include **nephrotoxicity** (kidney damage) and **ototoxicity** (damage to the ear).

## 4.1 Glycopeptide Antibiotics

Vancomycin is the most prominent member of a class of related antibiotics called glycopeptides. However, other less well-known glycopeptides are also clinically in use, and more glycopeptides continue to be discovered with every passing year.

The following is a list of clinically approved glycopeptides other than vancomycin [1]:

1. **Teicoplanin** is a natural product just like vancomycin. The clinically used teicoplanin antibiotic is a mixture of five lipoglycopeptide molecules differing in the length (C10-C11) and branching of the fatty acid tail. Teicoplanin has a much larger half-life (100–170 hours) compared to vancomycin (4–6 hours), as well as having better tissue penetration.
2. **Oritavancin** is a semisynthetic glycopeptide antibiotic and a derivative of a vancomycin analogue (chloroeremomycin). It has demonstrated activity *in vitro* against methicillin-resistant *S. aureus* MRSA and vancomycin-resistant enterococci (VRE), in both planktonic and biofilm states.
3. **Telavancin** is also a semisynthetic glycopeptide antibiotic and a direct derivative of vancomycin (effective against MRSA).
4. **Dalbavancin** is a semisynthetic derivative of the teicoplanin-like A40926 designed for use against vancomycin resistant organisms (effective against MRSA).

Together, glycopeptide antibiotics have somewhat eased the threat of methicillin-resistant *S. aureus* by giving clinicians several new drugs for its treatment.

## 4.2 Mechanism of Action

Vancomycin acts by binding to the cell wall and **inhibiting cell wall synthesis** in gram-positive bacteria (Fig. 4.3). It binds to the terminal (D-ala)-(D-ala) residues on the peptidoglycan precursor, competing with and preventing transpeptidase from binding and cross-linking peptides, thereby preventing complete cell wall formation.

Unfortunately, being a bulky molecule, vancomycin cannot easily pass through the outer membrane of gram-negative bacteria. It is therefore ineffective against gram-negative organisms except for some nongonococcal species of Neisseria.

### 4.2.1 Vancomycin Binds to the Cell Wall

Like penicillin, vancomycin does not lyse cells in the stationary phase. Unlike penicillin, Vancomycin **does not form protoplasts** [2]. Vancomycin has also been observed to inhibit the "growth" of *Streptococcus faecalis* protoplasts prepared using lysozyme [3]. This growth inhibition was observed using turbidometry.

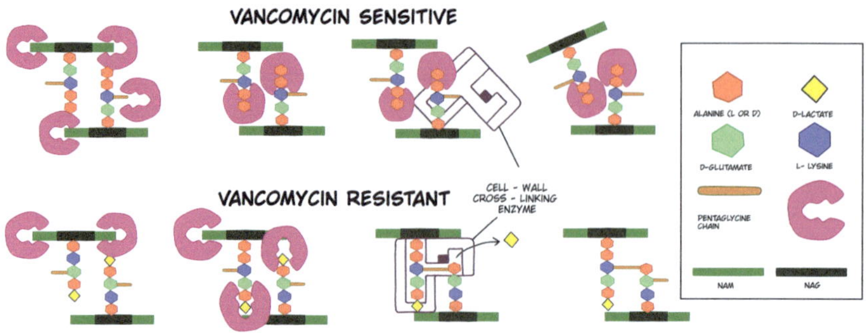


**Fig. 4.3** **(Above)** Vancomycin's mechanism of action. The antibiotic binds to terminal (D-ala)-(D-ala) residues, preventing transpeptidase from cross-linking peptides. **(Below)** One mechanism of vancomycin resistance. Bacterial strains with a terminal (D-ala) → (D-lactate) mutation are structurally incompatible with vancomycin and cannot be bound by it

These observations indicated that Vancomycin may have a different mechanism of action compared to penicillin, which forms and does not inhibit protoplasts. It also indicated that vancomycin's mechanism of action would have to be deciphered using a different set of experiments.

In an early experiment from 1965 [4], vancomycin was observed to bind to the cell wall using ***ex vivo*** **cell wall extracts**. To create a cell wall extract, bacteria were disrupted via sonication and centrifuged. The cell wall (white) was then carefully skimmed from the top of the pellet containing whole cells and other components (brown). Repeated centrifuging and washing steps coupled with chemical treatments to remove other unwanted components can eventually yield a highly pure cell wall extract. Proteins in particular had the potential to interfere with the downstream assay, as they absorb light at the same wavelength as vancomycin. Proteins were removed via trypsinization, where trypsin is added to hydrolyze proteins.

► **Remark**

Protoplasts cannot divide and therefore cannot grow in a conventional sense. However, protoplasts are still capable of **enlarging in size** while remaining **constant in numbers**. This volumetric growth can be tracked using turbidometry.

Vancomycin possesses a characteristic **absorption peak at 280 nm**. When mixed with this cell wall extract, the bound vancomycin concentration can easily be tracked spectrophotometrically. After allowing vancomycin to interact with the cell wall, unbound vancomycin can be removed by centrifuging at 12,100 g and discarding the supernatant (unbound vancomycin) and then resuspending the pellet and measuring absorbance (Fig. 4.4).

A more modern experiment can easily and elegantly confirm vancomycin/cell wall binding using **fluorescently labeled vancomycin** [5]. A fluorescent boron-dipyrromethene (**BODIPY**) tag can be covalently attached to the vancomycin

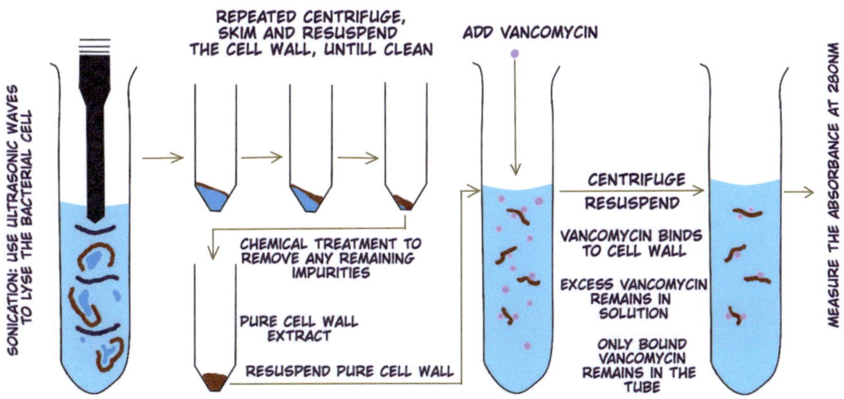


**Fig. 4.4** A 1965 experiment [4] to determine whether vancomycin binds to the bacterial cell wall. Detailed explanation in the text

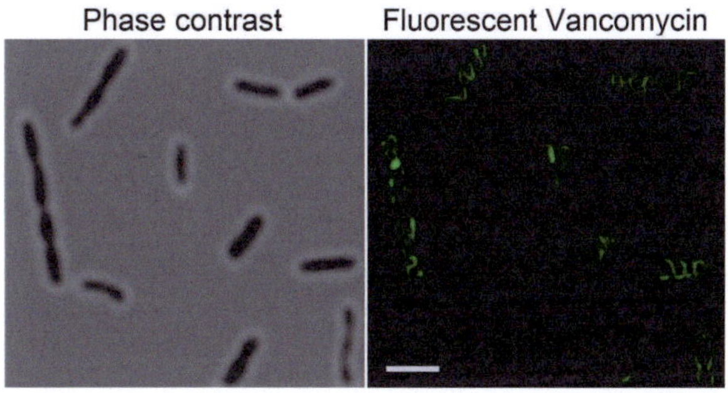


**Fig. 4.5** Fluorescent-tagged vancomycin localizing within the cell wall [5] (artist's impression). **(Left)** Phase contrast microscopy showing cellular morphology. **(Right)** Fluorescent microscopy showing BODIPY-vancomycin localization within the cell wall in a helical pattern. The scale bar represents 2 μm

molecule without affecting its antimicrobial properties. The subcellular localization of vancomycin can then be traced using fluorescent microscopy. Vancomycin was found to localize on the cell wall of *Bacillus subtilis* (PY79) in a **helical pattern** (Fig. 4.5), indicating a helical distribution of the peptidoglycan biosynthetic machinery. Although not performed in this experiment, colocalization of BODIPY-vancomycin with the cell wall can be confirmed by staining the latter with trypan blue or calcofluor white.

### 4.2.2 Vancomycin Binds to (D-ala)$_2$

Once vancomycin binding with peptidoglycan was established, peptidoglycan's constituent components could be assayed for binding against vancomycin one by

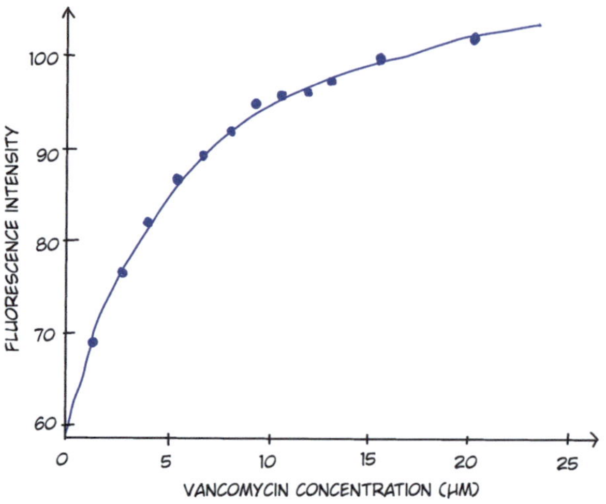


**Fig. 4.6** Fluorometric titration of a dansylated peptide containing (D-ala)-(D-ala) against unlabeled vancomycin. The fluorescence intensity of the resultant mixture increases proportionally with the amount of dansylated peptide added, confirming vancomycin binding

one till binding was detected. It was eventually found that vancomycin binds to the terminal (D-ala)-(D-ala) of the peptide component of the peptidoglycan precursor, acting like a transpeptidase analog (Infobox 4.2.3) and competing against the enzyme.

Vancomycin/(D-ala)-(D-ala) binding can be established using a simple fluorescence assay [6]. (L-lys)-(D-ala)-(D-ala) was tagged with **dansyl chloride**, a fluorophore that can be covalently linked to the free N-terminal (primary amine) of amino acids. Dansyl chloride is a **selectively fluorescent dye** that is sensitive to its immediate environment. Its fluorescence increases or decreases depending on the molecules that surround it. Therefore, if dansylated (L-lys)-(D-ala)-(D-ala) bound to vancomycin, we would expect to observe a change in fluorescence upon binding.

Figure 4.6 shows the expected results of the dansylated chloride binding titration. Here, small amounts of dansylated peptide were added incrementally to unbound vancomycin and the fluorescence was monitored after every step. The fluorescence increases proportionally with the amount of dansyl chloride added, confirming vancomycin binding.

### 4.2.3 Crystal Structure

X-ray crystallography is the least ambiguous, and usually final, method used to establish binding between two macromolecules. For vancomycin, a crystal of it in complex with (diacetyl lysine)-(D-ala)-(D-ala was obtained [7] (Fig. 4.7).

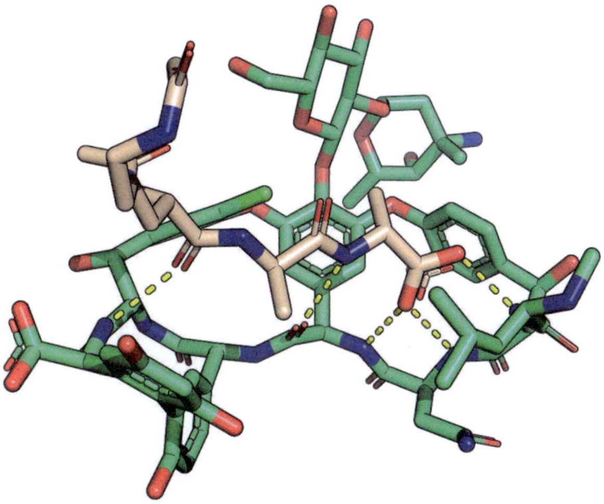

**Fig. 4.7** Crystal structure of a short peptide **(diacetyl lysine)-(D-ala)-(D-ala)** (beige) bound to **vancomycin** (green) through hydrogen bonds (yellow dotted lines). Oxygen atoms (hydrogen bond acceptors) are colored red. Nitrogen atoms (hydrogen bond donors) are colored blue. PDB ID: 1fvm [7]

From the structure, we can observe that vancomycin is able to form hydrogen bond interactions with the terminal (D-ala)-(D-ala) moieties of the NAM/NAG-peptides. Under normal circumstances, this is a five-point interaction.

**Infobox 4.1**

In some ways, vancomycin is the mirror opposite of penicillin. Penicillin is a small molecule with a molecular weight of **334.4 Da**. Vancomycin dwarfs it with a molecular weight of **1449 Da**.

Penicillin is a **substrate analog**. It mimics the structure of (D-ala)-(D-ala) which causes transpeptidase to irreversibly bind to it. Vancomycin is instead a **transpeptidase analog**. It competes with transpeptidase for (D-ala)-(D-ala) binding.

Given these complementary differences, the question arises: Will penicillin bind to vancomycin?

Interestingly enough this is indeed the case. Penicillin V (phenoxymethylpenicillin) binds to vancomycin [6] (Table 4.1). The interaction is a low affinity one, with an association constant ($K_A$) of only 0.11 $mM^{-1}$ (or a $K_D$ of 9 mM).

The binding affinity is low enough to be ignored when coadministering penicillin and vancomycin. They will not interact with each other *in vivo* at their therapeutic doses.

**Table 4.1** Association constants for binding of peptides to vancomycin

| Peptide | Association const. $K_A$ ($mM^{-1}$) |
|---|---|
| ADLAA | 300 |
| N,N'-Diacetyl-(L-Lys)-(D-ala)-(D-ala) | 1000–1500 |
| N,N'-Diacetyl-(L-Lys)-(D-ala)-(D-lactate) | 0.33 |
| N,N'-Diacetyl-(L-Lys)-(D-ala)-(D-alaninamide) | 2.8 |
| N-Acetyl-(D-ala)-(D-ala) | 16–20 |
| N-Acetyl-(D-ala) | 0.15–0.48 |
| N-Acetyl-(D-ala)-(L-Leu) | 0.089 |
| N-Acetyl-(L-ala)-(L-Leu) | 0.3–1.3 |
| Phenoxyacetyl-(D-ala)-(D-ala) | 210 |
| **Phenoxymethyl penicillin** | **0.11** |

## 4.3 Vancomycin Resistance Mechanisms

The evolution of resistance to vancomycin involves replacing the terminal D-ala in the peptidoglycan precursor with either D-lactate or D-serine [8] (Fig. 4.8). A **D-ala** → **D-lac** substitution causes the loss of one of the five hydrogen bonds normally present the vancomycin-peptide complex, greatly destabilizing it. A **D-ala** → **D-ser** substitution causes a steric clash with the peptide backbone of vancomycin, again destabilizing the complex. The D-lac mechanism of resistance is compared with vancomycin's mechanism of action in Fig. 4.3.

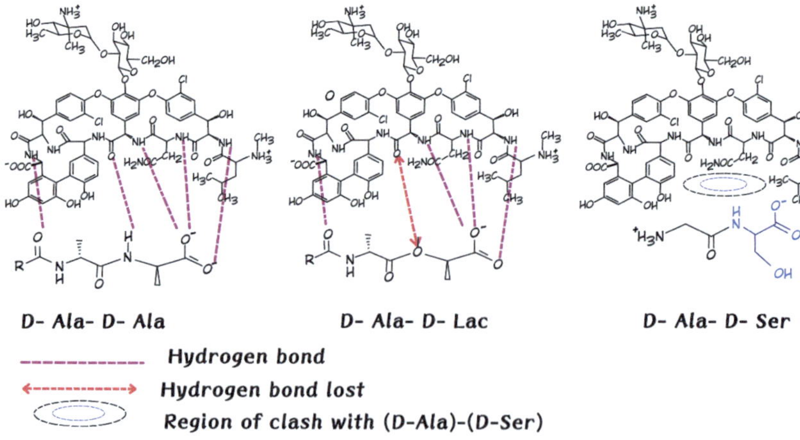


**Fig. 4.8** Amino acid substitutions on the terminal pentapeptide that cause vancomycin resistance

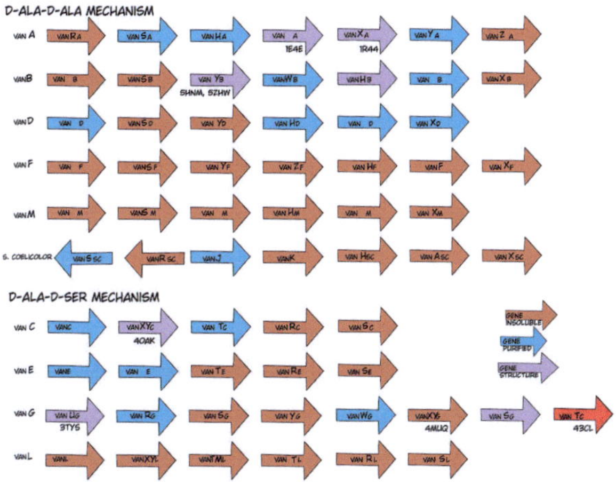


**Fig. 4.9** Known vancomycin resistance operons organized by mechanism type and then by the gene cassette name. **Key**: black outline = insoluble protein; tan = purified protein; dark green = crystal structure solved (PDB codes indicated under gene arrow). This figure is only presented for you to understand the magnitude of effort needed to change a single amino acid residue in a nonribosomally synthesized peptide

It should be noted that since the peptidoglycan precursor's pentapeptide is synthesized nonribosomally, these substitutions are not as trivial as point mutations on ribosomally synthesized peptides. Instead, entire metabolic pathways have to be evolved to make single amino acid modifications on the peptidoglycan precursor. This is why it took 30 years after the initial discovery of vancomycin for the first vancomycin resistant strains to be reported.

As of today, our understanding of the mechanisms and enzymes responsible for these two simple amino acid substitutions is still incomplete (Fig. 4.9).

## 4.4 Problems

### Problem 4.1

You have isolated an actinomycete from soil that you suspect secretes a vancomycin-like glycopeptide. You culture this organism in media that you expect is now rich with this glycopeptide. Design an experiment to purify the glycopeptide from media.

### Problem 4.2

You have set up a fluorometric titration of dansylated (L-lys)-(D-ala)-(D-ala) versus vancomycin exactly as described in the text (and in the reference [6]). You performed the assay and confirmed vancomycin binding to (D-ala)-(D-ala).

As soon as you finish your experiment, your guide interrupts you and gives you a new peptide he just finished synthesizing: (L-lys)-(D-selenoalanine)-(D-ala) [named lysela]. He suspects that despite the mutation, vancomycin will still bind to lysela.

Your guide wants results immediately, so you will have no time to dansylate lysela. You have to use your current experimental setup as is. Is there any simple modification you can make to your current experimental protocol to use it to measure vancomycin-lysela binding?

**Problem 4.3**

A bacterium gains vancomycin resistance by replacing the terminal (D-ala) on the peptidoglycan precursor with (D-lactate). Now vancomycin can no longer recognize the molecule. How does the bacterial transpeptidase still recognize the molecule and finish cross-linking the cell wall? This is an open question. You will need to find and read your own sources to attempt an answer.

## References

1. Binda E, Marinelli F, Marcone GL (2014) Old and new glycopeptide antibiotics: action and resistance. Antibiotics 3(4):572–594
2. Jordan DC, Reynolds PE (1967) Vancomycin. In: Mechanism of action. Springer, pp 102–116
3. Shockman GD, Lampen JO (1962) Inhibition by antibiotics of the growth of bacterial and yeast protoplasts. J Bacteriol 84(3):508–512
4. Best GK (1965) Mechanism of action of vancomycin. PhD thesis, Oklahoma State University
5. Muchová K, Wilkinson AJ, Barák I (2011) Changes of lipid domains in bacillus subtilis cells with disrupted cell wall peptidoglycan. FEMS Microbiol Lett 325(1):92–98
6. Popieniek PH, Pratt RF (1987) A fluorescent ligand for binding studies with glycopeptide antibiotics of the vancomycin class. Analyt Biochem 165(1):108–113
7. Nitanai Y, Kikuchi T, Kakoi K, Hanamaki S, Fujisawa I, Aoki K (2009) Crystal structures of the complexes between vancomycin and cell-wall precursor analogs. J Mol Biol 385(5):1422–1432
8. Stogios PJ, Savchenko A (2020) Molecular mechanisms of vancomycin resistance. Protein Sci 29(3):654–669

# Antimicrobial Peptides

# 5

Deepesh Nagarajan

**Abstract**

Antimicrobial peptides (AMPs) are a diverse group of peptides that evolved across all kingdoms of life. Gramicidin, daptomycin, bacitracin, and colistin are notable examples of clinically used AMPs. Antimicrobial peptides are attracted to negatively charged bacterial membranes via coulombic attraction. AMPs disrupt the cell membrane via mechanisms described as the carpet model, toroidal pore model, and barrel stave model. The membrane disruptions formed will lead to the exudation of cytoplasmic contents and the death of the bacterium. Membrane localization can be observed via fluorescence microscopy involving the use of fluorescently tagged AMPs. Scanning electron microscopy (SEM) and transmission electron microscopy (TEM) can be used to visualize membrane damage caused by AMP. Simple radioassays can be used to track small-molecule leakage from the bacterial cytoplasm. Secondary metabolic inhibitory effects of AMPs also contribute to their mechanism of action. Resistance mechanisms to AMPs include proteolytic enzymes, changing the membrane charge, formation of biofilms, and the use of multidrug efflux pumps.

**Keywords**

Antimicrobial peptides · Amphiphile · Membrane-acting · Fluorescence microscopy · Antibiotic resistance

---

D. Nagarajan (✉)
Department of Biotechnology, M.S. Ramaiah University of Applied Sciences, Bangalore, India

Department of Microbiology, St. Xavier's College, Mumbai, India
e-mail: deepeshn.bt.ls@msruas.ac.in; deepesh.nagarajan@xaviers.edu

© The Editor(s) (if applicable) and The Author(s), under exclusive license to Springer Nature Singapore Pte Ltd. 2024

D. Nagarajan (ed.), *Antibiotics and Their Mechanisms of Action*,
https://doi.org/10.1007/978-981-97-6851-6_5

Antimicrobial peptides (AMPs) are a diverse group of antibacterial compounds that have an ancient evolutionary origin and are produced across all kingdoms of life, ranging from soil bacteria to humans.

## 5.1 History

The therapeutic potential of antimicrobial peptides was first realized in 1939, when **René J. Dubos** discovered **gramicidin**, an antibacterial agent that inhibits the growth of gram-positive bacteria. It was the first antibiotic to be tested clinically, and it was used in topical form to treat wounds and ulcers during World War II.

The next important development in the field was the discovery of polymyxins, discovered independently by three laboratories in 1947. The most important polymyxin, **colistin** (polymyxin E), was discovered in Japan in 1949 by **Y. Koyama**. Koyama isolated colistin from a flask of fermenting *Bacillus polymyxa* var. colistinus. It has been available since 1959 for the treatment of infections caused by gram-negative bacteria. Polymyxins represent a significant advancement over gramicidins because they can be administered internally without causing hemolysis.

There are two forms of colistin available commercially: colistin sulfate and colistimethate sodium. **Colistin sulfate** is used in topical preparations for the treatment of bacterial skin infections or administered orally in the form of tablets or syrup for bowel decontamination. **Colistimethate sodium** is the injectable form and is an inactive prodrug. It is readily hydrolyzed to a variety of active methanesulfonate derivatives.

A third and final wave of interest in AMPs began in 1987 with the isolation of **magainin** from the skin of the African clawed frog (**Xenopus laevis**) [1] (Fig. 5.1). Its discoverer, **Michael Zasloff**, was impressed with the frog's ability to resist infection after invasive surgery even when placed in a non-sterile tank. He created a skin extract and fractionated it using ion-exchange chromatography on carboxymethyl cellulose. He discovered magainin after carefully analyzing the fractions that showed bacterial inhibition on a lawn of *E. coli*. Shortly thereafter magainin was rationally improved to create **Pexiganan**. Pexiganan unfortunately failed clinical trials on patients with diabetic foot ulcers, as it was no better than existing treatments.

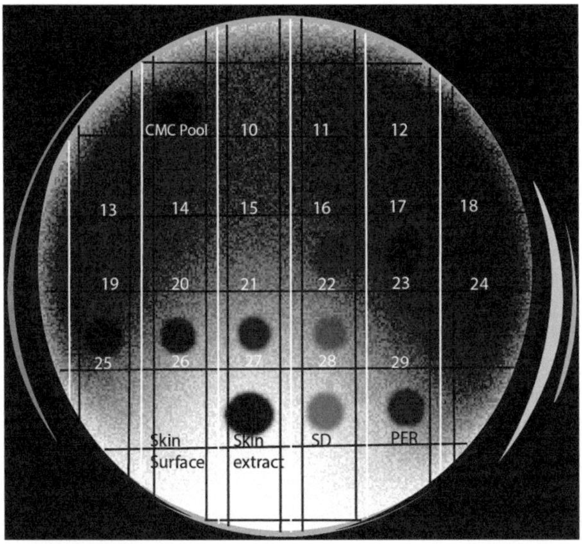


**Fig. 5.1** A crude magainin extract inhibits a lawn of *Escherichia coli* (artist's impression). Each cell represents a fraction isolated using ion-exchange chromatography on carboxymethyl cellulose. Fractions 22–28 all show the presence of magainin

In many ways Pexiganan characterizes the third wave of AMPs. Many promising peptides have been developed, yet **none have passed clinical trials** for a variety of reasons. Nevertheless researchers are learning from past mistakes and pressing on with improved molecules.

## 5.2 Common Chemical Characteristics

Despite being an incredibly diverse group of molecules, AMPs share some common structural traits:

1. All are **short** peptide molecules ($\leq$ 20 residues). Larger AMPs are merely proteins and cannot easily be secreted by organisms.
2. Usually **positively charged**. The positive charge is necessary to interact with the negatively charged bacterial cell membrane. It should be noted that neutral and negatively charged AMPs also exist.
3. **Amphipathic**. Amphipathicity allows the peptide to remain soluble in aqueous solvents and the bacterial membrane.
4. Either **cyclic** or possess **N-/C-terminal "caps"** (nonprotein chemical moieties). Exposed N-/C-terminals are easy targets for hydrolysis and degradation.
5. Incorporate **noncanonical** and **D-amino acids** into their sequence, possibly to make them harder targets for degradation.

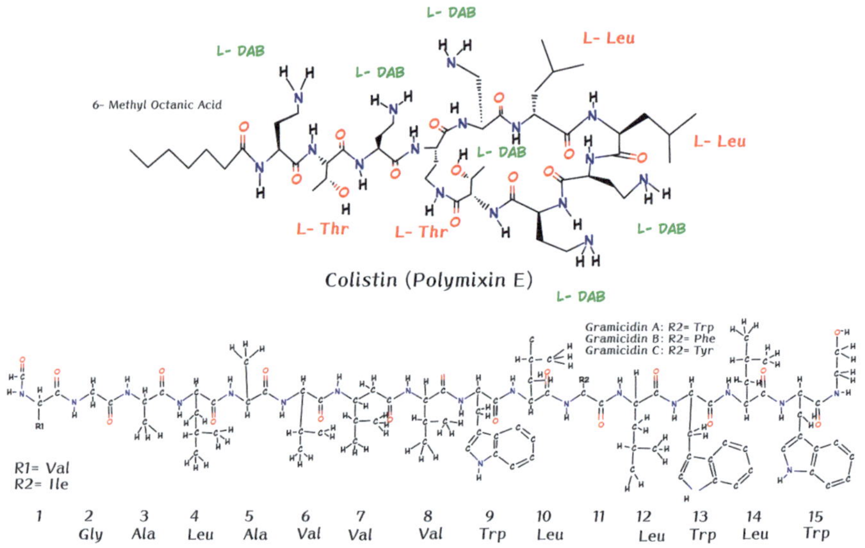


**Fig. 5.2** The structures of colistin and gramicidin are presented as representative AMPs. **Colistin** is short, positively charged, amphiphilic, and cyclic, possesses noncanonical amino acid residues (L-DAB = diaminobutyric acid), and also possesses an N-terminal cap (6-methyl octanoic acid). **Gramicidin** is short, neutral, mostly hydrophobic, and linear, possesses only natural amino acids, and also possesses N-/C-terminal caps. Both are effective AMPs when used correctly

The aforementioned characteristics are a rule of thumb (much like Lipinski's rules) and not a natural or a biophysical constraint. AMPs exist that violate some or even most of these rules (Fig. 5.2).

## 5.3 Clinically Used AMPs

Despite the number of discovered AMPs ranging in the tens of thousands, only a handful has made it to clinical use.

1. **Gramicidins A, B, C**: used to treat infected wounds and as eye drops*
2. **Gramicidin S**: infected wounds*
3. **Colistin/Polymyxin E**: drug of last resort for gram-negative carbapenem-resistant infections. It causes nephrotoxicity
4. **Daptomycin**: drug of last resort for gram-positive carbapenem-resistant infections. Numerous side effects (edema—swelling of ankles and feet, eosinophilia, and dyspnea—shortness of breath)
5. **Bacitracin/Polymyxin B**: topical agents for minor injuries*. Components of neosporin along with neomycin

*: topical agents only. They cause fatal hemolysis, nephrotoxicity, and hepatotoxicity if used internally.

AMPs are highly **toxic**. From the list above, it is apparent that most cause fatal hemolysis and are for external use only. The AMPs that can be used internally still cause nephrotoxicity or a host of other side effects.

AMPs are still clinically relevant as they can **treat drug-resistant infections**. Evolving resistance against them is extremely hard for pathogens due to their mechanism of action. Given these facts, they are termed as **drugs of last resort**.

## 5.4 Mechanisms of Action

AMPs bind to and localize within the bacterial cell membrane. Positively charged AMPs do so through coulombic interactions, and other AMPs do so through other mechanisms.

Once incorporated, they **disrupt the cell membrane** causing large-scale membrane damage and exudation of cytoplasmic contents (**carpet model**, Fig. 5.3).

Alternatively, AMPs can form **nanometer-scale pores** on the cell membrane, causing the leakage of cytoplasmic small molecules and ultimately death (**barrel stave model**, Fig. 5.4, and the closely related **toroidal pore model**).

Since there are tens of thousands of known AMPs, these models are only generalizations. The specific mechanisms of individual AMPs may differ from these templates. The mechanisms of the same AMP may even differ between strains.

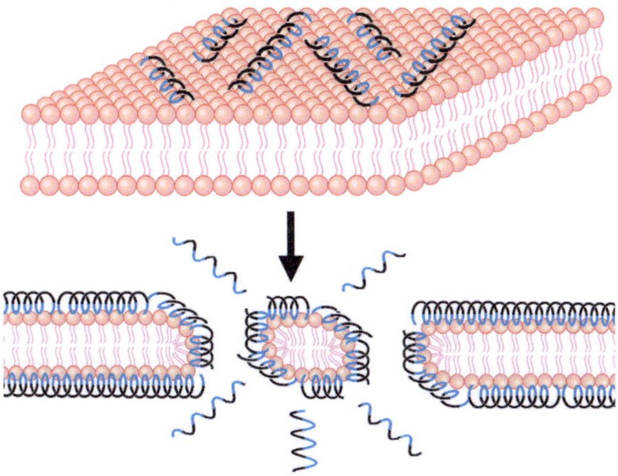

**Fig. 5.3** In the **carpet model**, the peptides disrupt the membrane by orienting parallel to the surface of the lipid bilayer and forming an extensive layer or carpet. Hydrophilic regions of the peptide are shown colored red, and hydrophobic regions of the peptide are shown colored blue

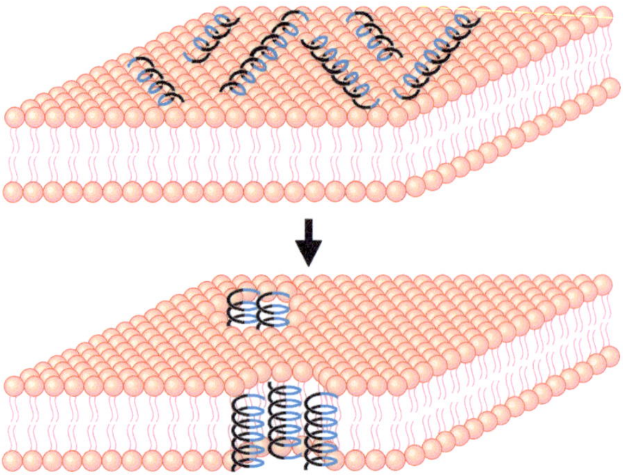

**Fig. 5.4** In the **barrel stave** model, the attached peptides aggregate and insert into the membrane bilayer so that the hydrophobic peptide regions align with the lipid core region and the hydrophilic peptide regions form the interior region of the pore

### 5.4.1 Membrane Localization

AMP localization within the bacterial membrane can be confirmed using fluorescent dyes such as Fluorescein isothiocyanate (**FITC**). FITC can be covalently linked to any peptide as an N-terminus "cap." Other counter-dyes can stain the bacterial chromosome (4',6-diamidino-2-phenylindole—**DAPI**) and cell membrane (**Nile red**) of a given pathogen.

All dyes can be simultaneously visualized using confocal or apotome fluorescent microscopy.

If FITC colocalizes with the membrane and not the nucleus, then the AMP in question is a membrane-binding agent (Fig. 5.5 [2]).

### 5.4.2 Membrane Disruption

Large-scale membrane disruptions can easily be visualized using **scanning electron microscopy** (SEM), **transmission electron microscopy** (TEM), or **atomic force microscopy** (AFM).

Membrane disruption causes the **Exudation** of cytoplasmic contents and **blebbing**: the formation of small, detached "bubbles" of cell membrane.

Membrane disruption cannot directly be visualized for gram-positive organisms using SEM or AFM because of their thick cell walls. However, protoplasts can be created, and the cell membrane, along with any disruptions induced upon it, can then be directly observed (Fig. 5.6 [3]).

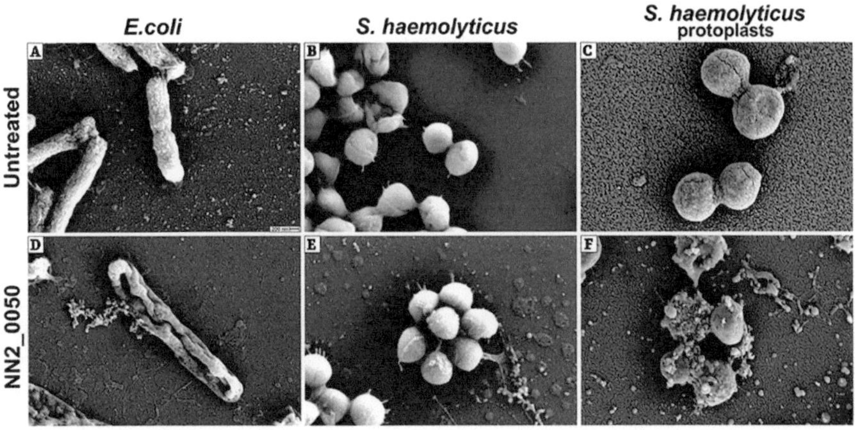


**Fig. 5.5 Scanning electron microscopy** (SEM) with NN2_0050, an experimental AMP [3]. (**a**) Untreated *E. coli* cells observed under ×50,000 magnification. (**d**) *E. coli* cells treated with NN2_0050. Membrane disruption and exudation of cytoplasmic contents, including the bacterial chromosome, is apparent. (**b**) Untreated *Staphylococcus haemolyticus* cells observed under ×50,000 magnification. (**e**) *S. haemolyticus* cells treated with NN2_0050, displaying some exudation of cytoplasmic contents. (**c**) Untreated *S. haemolyticus* protoplasts observed under ×50,000 magnification. (**f**) *S. haemolyticus* protoplasts treated with NN2_0050 observed under ×50,000 magnification. Blebbing is easily observable on all cell membranes. Detached blebs are also observable around protoplasts as small spheres

TEM does not suffer from this drawback as all bacterial samples are cut into nanometer-thick sections before visualizing, allowing us to observe all cellular components simultaneously (Fig. 5.7 [4]).

### 5.4.3 Pore Formation

Nanometer-scale pores cannot be visualized using most microscopic techniques. However, the loss of cytoplasmic small molecules they cause can easily be tracked using appropriate **small-molecule tracers**. If these tracers are observed to leak out of cells upon the introduction of an AMP and if large-scale membrane disruption is not observed, then the existence of nanoscale pores can be inferred.

Tracers can easily be introduced into the bacterial cell via passive diffusion. Typically incubation with a tracer at 8°C overnight (to suspend metabolism) will be sufficient. Smaller molecules are preferred over larger ones simply because they can diffuse across membranes more easily.

▶ **Remark**
Although uranium is a radioactive element, it cannot be used as a radiotracer due to its extremely long half-life.

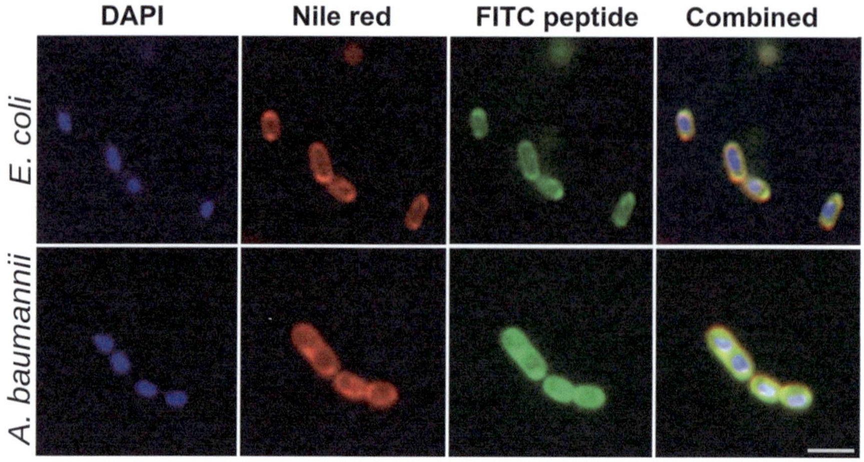


| Culture | R/G | G/B | R/B |
|---|---|---|---|
| *E. coli* | **0.46** | −0.20 | −0.24 |
| *A. baumannii* | **0.65** | −0.22 | −0.06 |

| | | |
|---|---|---|
| R | (RED channel) | Nile red stain |
| G | (GREEN channel) | FITC-labeled peptide |
| B | (BLUE channel) | DAPI stain |

**Fig. 5.6** **Fluorescent confocal microscopy** with **Ω76**: an experimental AMP [2]. **(Top)** FITC-labeled Ω76-treated *E. coli*. Ω76 colocalized with Nile red, indicating a membrane-binding propensity. **(Bottom)** FITC-labeled Ω76-treated *Acinetobacter baumannii*. Ω76 again colocalized with Nile red, indicating a membrane-binding propensity. **(Table)** Pearson's correlation coefficients given for all combinations of stains (DAPI/FITC peptide/Nile red). Better stain colocalization is denoted by higher correlation values. In both cases, the Nile red/FITC peptide pair was the most strongly correlated. Scale bar = 2 μm

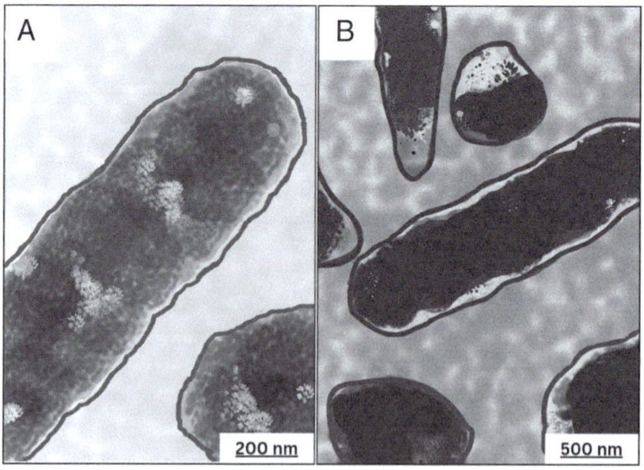


**Fig. 5.7** **Transmission electron microscopy** (TEM) of *E. coli* treated with **gramicidin** (artist's impression). **(a)** Micrograph of untreated *E. coli*. **(b)** After treatment with gramicidin, showing loss of inner membrane integrity

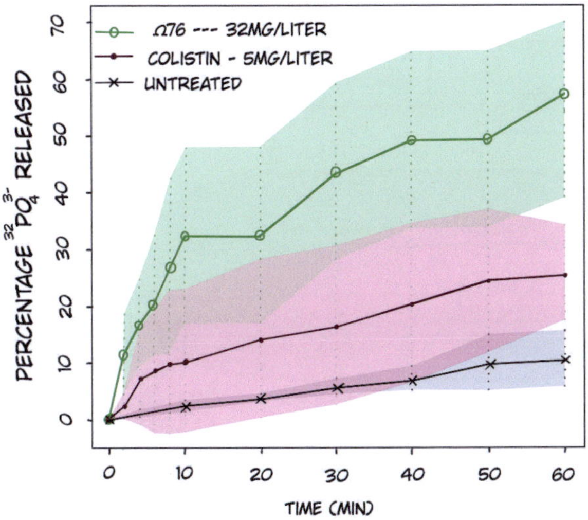


**Fig. 5.8** $^{32}$**P** radioassay showing pore formation for Ω76 [5, 2] and colistin sulfate on *A. baumannii*. Both AMPs did not cause large-scale membrane disruption on this strain. Error bars indicate standard deviations for three replicates

Tracers may be:

1. **Elemental**: Ideally elements with no biological role that are expected to be absent in both the organism and buffer. Salts of **osmium**, **tungstate**, or **uranyl** can be used. These salts are also used for staining of TEM samples and should be easily available. Quantification is performed using **mass spectrometry** (preferably ICP-MS).
2. **Radioactive**: Soluble forms of any $\alpha$- or $\beta$-emitter will suffice. $^{32}$**P** and $^{35}$**S** are recommended as their acids are extremely affordable. Quantification is performed using **scintillation counting**.

Cells imbibed with an appropriate small molecule can then be resuspended in saline and mixed with AMP. The saline can then be separated via centrifugation or millipore filtration and assayed for tracer.

An AMP that forms pores would be expected to cause cells to release tracer into its surrounding medium over time (Fig. 5.8 [5, 2]).

## 5.4.4 Metabolic Inhibition

Although the formation of transmembrane pores and extensive membrane damage eventually leads to the lysis of microbial cells, there is increasing speculation that these effects are not the only mechanisms of microbial killing [6]. There is

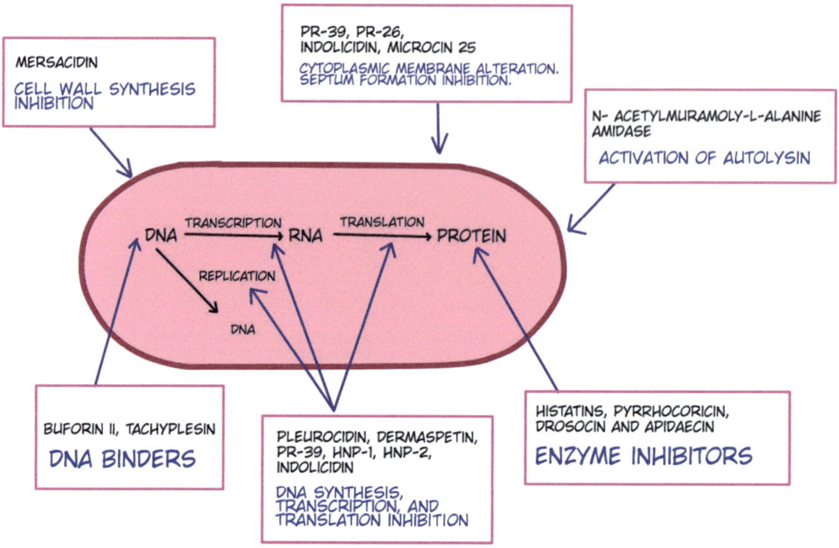


**Fig. 5.9** AMPs work through multiple mechanisms of action

increasing evidence to indicate that antimicrobial peptides have other intracellular targets including but not limited to inhibition of cytoplasmic membrane **septum formation**, inhibition of **cell wall synthesis**, inhibition of **nucleic acid synthesis**, inhibition of **protein synthesis**, and inhibition of **enzymatic activity** (Fig. 5.9).

A comprehensive description of the experiments performed to determine all these mechanisms of action is beyond the scope of this textbook and is only mentioned to convey to the reader the immense scope of this subject.

## 5.5 AMP Resistance Mechanisms

They include [7] (Fig. 5.10):

1. **Proteolysis** of AMPs by secreted, membrane bound, or cytosolic **proteases**
2. **Electrostatic repulsion**. By replacing the cell membrane's negative charge with a positive one, pathogens can prevent positively charged AMPs from binding.
3. **Biofilms** and exopolymers: exopolysaccharides (EPS) and capsular polysaccharides (CPS). A thick biopolymer coating will place ample distance between the cell wall and AMPs.
4. **Alteration of the pentapeptide** amino acid composition to evade AMPs that bind to the cell wall, in a manner very similar to resistance mechanisms against vancomycin (read Sect. 4.3 for more details).

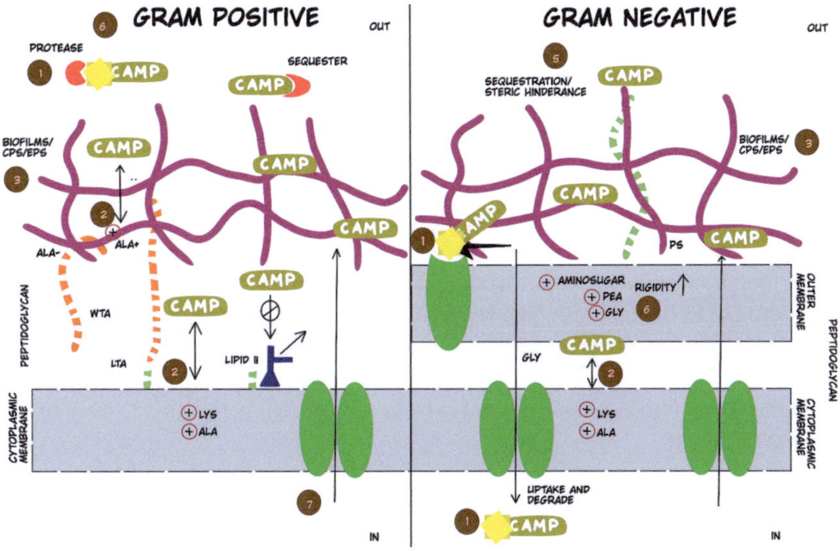


**Fig. 5.10** The multiple resistance mechanism pathogens adopt to combat AMPs [7]. Mechanisms in **gram-positive** bacteria are on the left. Mechanisms in **gram-negative** bacteria are on the right. Details on resistance mechanisms are provided in the text. **CAMP** = cationic antimicrobial peptide. Numbers depict the mechanisms described in this section

5. Sequestration or **steric hindrance** by O-antigen lipopolysaccharide (LPS). Long sugar chains extending out of the outer membrane can form a barrier that prevents AMPs from interacting with it and the cell membrane.
6. Enhanced **rigidity** of the outer membrane by lipid A acylation prevents AMP insertion into the lipid bilayer.
7. **Efflux pumps** for AMPs that have cytoplasmic targets. Read Sect. 3.4.3 for more details.

## 5.6 Problems

### Problem 5.1

Your colleague is working on an AMP. It is effective against *S. aureus* both *in vitro* and *in vivo*. She incubates *S. aureus* with AMP, centrifuges it down, then mounts, and treats it for scanning electron microscopy using standard protocols. Unfortunately, the surface of the bacteria appears intact.

Do these observations indicate that the cell membrane of *S. aureus* is not affected by this AMP? (yes/no)
If you answered no, then describe two experiments that would help your colleague observe the effect of the AMP on the cell membrane of *S. aureus*.

**Problem 5.2**

You have performed two experiments with your AMP on *E. coli*:

1. Fluorescent confocal microscopy: You observed that your AMP colocalizes with DAPI but not with Nile red.
2. Scanning electron microscopy: You observed large-scale membrane damage.

Do these experiments indicate that membrane damage is the direct cause of cell death? Explain.

**Problem 5.3**

Design a radioassay that can be used to detect and quantify the leakage of the bacterial chromosome from a culture treated with an AMP.

**Problem 5.4**

Your guide hands you a pathogenic strain that is resistant to all the AMPs he tested it on. After some experimentation, he has narrowed down its mechanism of resistance to three possibilities:

1. Secretion of extracellular nonspecific protease
2. Secretion of capsular polysaccharides
3. Electrostatic repulsion caused by an accumulation of positively charged groups on the cell membrane

Design a series of experiments to determine which of these mechanisms are responsible for AMP resistance. Note that two or more mechanisms could operate simultaneously.

## References


1. Zasloff M (1987) Magainins, a class of antimicrobial peptides from Xenopus skin: isolation, characterization of two active forms, and partial cDNA sequence of a precursor. Proc Natl Acad Sci 84(15):5449–5453
2. Nagarajan D, Roy N, Kulkarni O, Nanajkar N, Datey A, Ravichandran S, Thakur C, Aprameya IV, Sarma SP, Chakravortty D, et al. (2019) $\omega$76: A designed antimicrobial peptide to combat carbapenem- and tigecycline-resistant *Acinetobacter baumannii*. Sci Adv 5(7):eaax1946
3. Nagarajan D, Nagarajan T, Roy N, Kulkarni O, Ravichandran S, Mishra M, Chakravortty D, Chandra N (2018) Computational antimicrobial peptide design and evaluation against multidrug-resistant clinical isolates of bacteria. J Biol Chem 293(10):3492–3509

4. Hartmann M, Berditsch M, Hawecker J, Ardakani MF, Gerthsen D, Ulrich AS (2010) Damage of the bacterial cell envelope by antimicrobial peptides gramicidin A and PGLa as revealed by transmission and scanning electron microscopy. Antimicrobial Agents Chemotherapy 54(8):3132–3142
5. Nanajkar N, Mruthyunjaya LS, Nagarajan D (2023) A simple radioassay to detect nanoscale membrane disruption. Methods Protocols 6(2):23
6. Brogden KA (2005) Antimicrobial peptides: pore formers or metabolic inhibitors in bacteria? Nature Rev Microbiol 3(3):238–250
7. Joo H-S, Fu C-I, Otto M (2016) Bacterial strategies of resistance to antimicrobial peptides. Phil Trans Royal Soc B Biol Sci 371(1695):20150292

# Quinolones

# 6

Deepesh Nagarajan

**Abstract**

Quinolones are antibiotics that share a bicyclic core structure related to 4-quinolone. Quinolones have been developed over four generations, with drugs ranging from nalidixic acid to ciprofloxacin and trovafloxacin available for clinical use. Quinolones inhibit DNA replication by binding to bacterial type II topoisomerase (DNA gyrase), thereby preventing it from relaxing supercoiled chromosomal DNA. A radioassay involving the use of $^{14}C$ thymine, $^{14}C$ uracil, and $^{14}C$ arginine can be used to determine whether nalidixic acid inhibits DNA replication, transcription, or translation, respectively. Agarose gel electrophoresis can be used to determine whether ciprofloxacin inhibits the activity of gyrase on supercoiled plasmid *in vitro*. The X-ray crystallographic structure of quinolone-bound gyrase reveals that $\pi$-$\pi$ stacking interactions and coordination with magnesium mediate this interaction.

**Keywords**

Quinolone · Gyrase · Supercoiling · Antibiotic resistance

Quinolones are a large group of antibiotics that are united by a shared bicyclic core structure related to the substance 4-quinolone (Fig. 6.1).

D. Nagarajan (✉)
Department of Biotechnology, M.S. Ramaiah University of Applied Sciences, Bangalore, India

Department of Microbiology, St. Xavier's College, Mumbai, India
e-mail: deepeshn.bt.ls@msruas.ac.in; deepesh.nagarajan@xaviers.edu

© The Editor(s) (if applicable) and The Author(s), under exclusive license to Springer Nature Singapore Pte Ltd. 2024
D. Nagarajan (ed.), *Antibiotics and Their Mechanisms of Action*,
https://doi.org/10.1007/978-981-97-6851-6_6

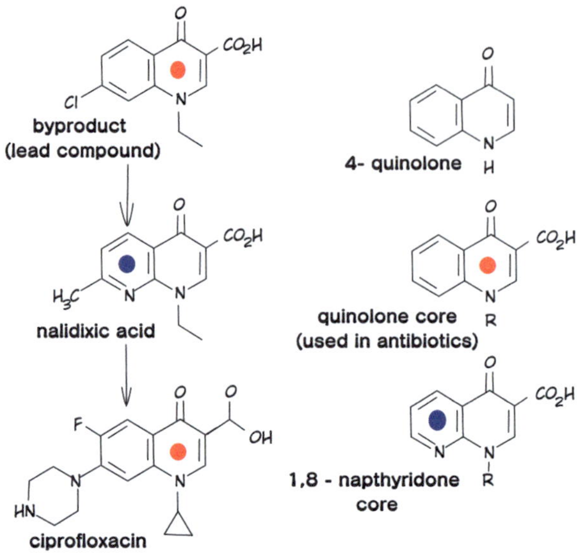


**Fig. 6.1** The original by-product tested for antibacterial activity by **George Lesher**. Note that this by-product possessed a **quinolone** core. **Nalidixic acid** was developed from this lead, and it possessed superior antimicrobial properties. Note that nalidixic acid possesses a **1,8-naphthyridone** core. Note that nalidixic acid is still considered to be a quinolone despite not possessing a quinolone core. **Ciprofloxacin** was developed from nalidixic acid and reverted back to a **quinolone** core. Ciprofloxacin is still in widespread clinical use today, whereas nalidixic acid has been relegated to niche roles. The reason for the **quinolone→1,8-naphthyridone→quinolone** flip-flop during drug development of this class has never been fully understood [1]

## 6.1 History

The progenitor of the quinolone class was discovered by **George Lesher** working at **Sterling Drug Inc.** in 1962 as a by-product during the synthesis of antimalarial quinine compounds. It demonstrated anti-gram-negative antibacterial activity, but its potency and antimicrobial spectrum were not significant enough to be useful in therapy. Building on this lead, **nalidixic acid** was synthesized and commercialized (Fig. 6.1). It should be noted that researchers at **Imperial Chemical Industries** independently reported quinolone core antibacterials as early as 1960 [1].

Nalidixic acid was further developed into the **fluoroquinolone** class, chief among them being **ciprofloxacin**. Ciprofloxacin is one of the most commonly used antibiotics today.

## 6.2 Classes of Quinolones

The quinolones can be divided into four generations of drugs based on their expanding spectrum of activity [2]. The quinolones can be differentiated within classes based on their pharmacokinetic properties. It should be noted that as this class is still developing, different authors will present different classification schemes.

1. First-generation quinolones (e.g., nalidixic acid) have narrow spectrums (gram-negative only) and achieve minimal serum levels.
2. Second-generation quinolones (e.g., ciprofloxacin) have increased gram-negative and systemic activity.
3. Third-generation quinolones (e.g., levofloxacin) have expanded activity against gram-positive bacteria and atypical pathogens.
4. Fourth-generation quinolones (e.g., trovafloxacin) add significant activity against anaerobes.

A more detailed description of quinolones can be found in Table 6.1.

**Table 6.1** List and description of quinolone generations, as described by King et al. [2]

| Generation | Examples | Spectrum of activity | Clinical indications |
|---|---|---|---|
| First | Nalidixic acid, cinoxacin | Gram-negative organisms (but not *Pseudomonas spp.*). | Uncomplicated UTIs |
| Second | Ciprofloxacin, norfloxacin, lomefloxacin, enoxacin, ofloxacin | Gram-negative organisms (including *Pseudomonas spp.*), some gram-positive organisms (including *Staphylococcus aureus* but not *Streptococcus pneumoniae*), and some atypical pathogens | Uncomplicated and complicated UTIs and pyelonephritis, STDs, prostatitis, skin, and soft tissue infections |
| Third | levofloxacin, sparfloxacin, gatifloxacin, moxifloxacin | The same as for second-generation agents plus expanded gram-positive coverage (penicillin-sensitive and penicillin-resistant *S. pneumoniae*) and expanded activity against atypical pathogens | Acute exacerbations of chronic bronchitis, community-acquired pneumonia |
| Fourth | Trovafloxacin | The same as for third-generation agents plus broad anaerobic coverage | The same as for first-, second-, and third-generation agents (excluding complicated urinary tract infections and pyelonephritis) plus intra-abdominal infections, nosocomial pneumonia, pelvic infections |

Quinolones are generally safe with few adverse side effects reported. The most common adverse effects of the fluoroquinolones are nausea, vomiting, and diarrhea, which occur in 3–6 percent of recipients. Third-generation quinolones onward display some rare but serious side effects:

1. **Central nervous system effects**: headache, confusion, and dizziness
2. **Phototoxicity** or damage to the skin upon exposure to UV light, more common with lomefloxacin and sparfloxacin
3. **Cardiotoxicity**, associated with sparfloxacin
4. **Hepatotoxicity**, associated with trovafloxacin

## 6.3 Mechanism of Action

Quinolones **inhibit DNA replication** by binding to the bacterial type II topoisomerase (**DNA gyrase**) and preventing it from relaxing supercoiled chromosomal DNA.

### 6.3.1 Type II Topoisomerase

Before proceeding, it is essential to recollect what DNA supercoiling is and why enzymes are needed to "relax" DNA (Fig. 6.2).

Very briefly, as the double helix is unwound during replication, tension (or **positive supercoils**) builds up at the front of the replication fork. Once DNA becomes too tense (or too positively supercoiled), it cannot be unwound any further. Topoisomerases are therefore needed to "relax" (or **reduce positive supercoiling**) the double helix and allow the replication fork to move forward.

Type II topoisomerases relieve tension (or reduce positive supercoiling) by cleaving a double strand of DNA, passing it over another double strand, and then joining back the broken strand. This cleavage requires ATP and **removes two positive supercoils** (or introduces two negative supercoils).

## 6.4 Inhibition of DNA Replication

**DNA replication**, **RNA polymerization**, and **protein synthesis** in the presence and absence of nalidixic acid were tracked and quantified using a simple series of experiments involving radiolabeled small molecules [4].

DNA replication was very simply quantified using $^{14}C$-labeled thymine as a tracker. *Escherichia coli* was inoculated into **minimal media** containing **no other source of thymine**. Two such flasks of minimal media in the presence of the radiotracker were prepared: the treated and control. At the start of the experiment, an inhibitory concentration of **Nalidixic acid** was added to the **test** but **not to the control**. At 10 minute intervals and for both flasks, aliquots were pipetted out, and

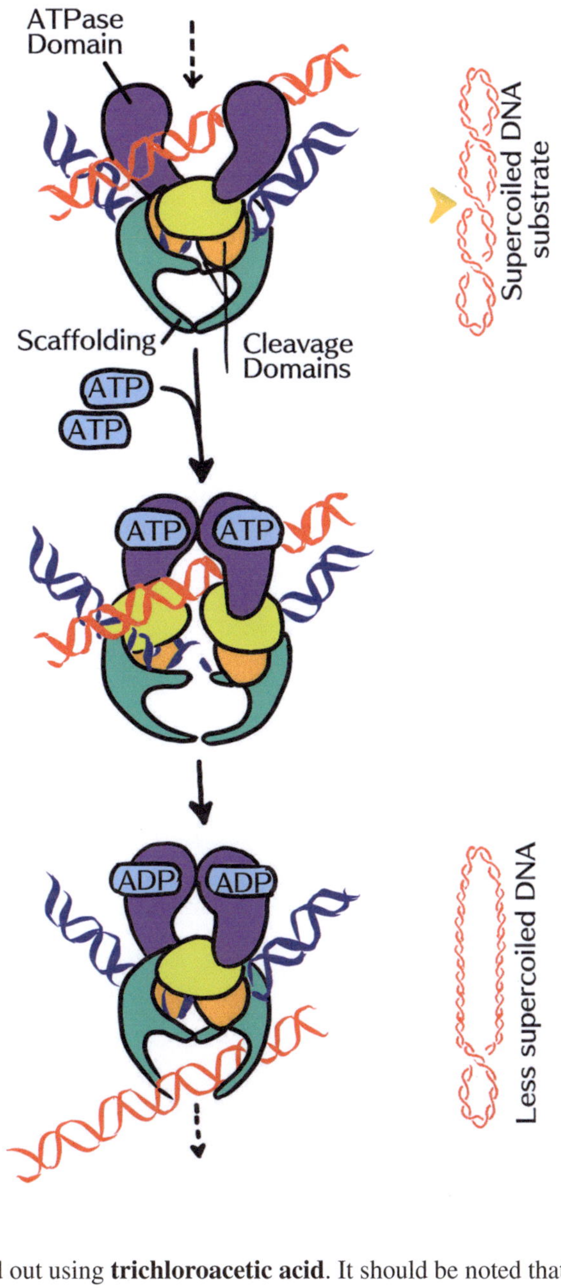


**Fig. 6.2** Mechanism of action for type II topoisomerases (DNA gyrases) [3]

their **DNA was precipitated** out using **trichloroacetic acid**. It should be noted that trichloroacetic acid precipitates all macromolecules (DNA, RNA, and proteins); however in this case only the DNA will be radioactive. The radioactivity of the precipitate was measured using **scintillation counting**.

**Table 6.2** Three experiments to determine the effect of quinolones (nalidixic acid) on DNA, RNA, and protein synthesis

| Experiment | Media substrates |
|---|---|
| DNA replication TREATED | $^{14}$C-labeled thymine nalidixic acid |
| DNA replication CONTROL | $^{14}$C-labeled thymine |
| RNA polymerization TREATED | $^{14}$C-labeled uracil nalidixic acid |
| RNA polymerization CONTROL | $^{14}$C-labeled uracil |
| protein synthesis TREATED | $^{14}$C-labeled L-arginine nalidixic acid |
| protein-synthesis CONTROL | $^{14}$C-labeled L-arginine |

Three separate experiments to quantify the effect of nalidixic acid on the aforementioned three macromolecules were performed (Table 6.2), with a treated and control condition each:

**Proposed experiment 6.1**

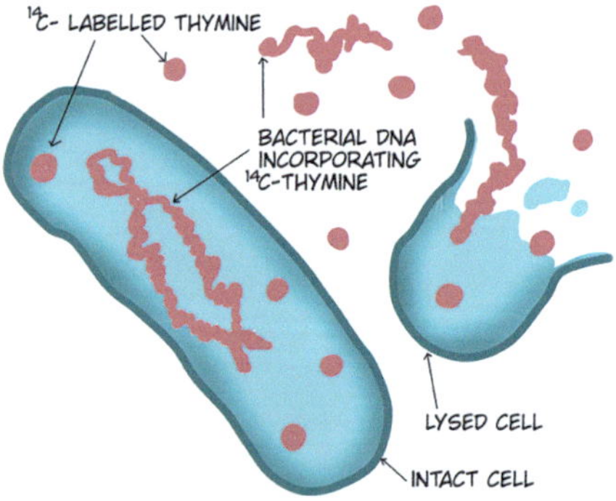


Why do we use trichloroacetic acid to precipitate DNA?

Would not it be simpler to **centrifuge the cells**, discard the supernatant, and assay the **radioactivity of the pellet only**?

**No**, actually.

The culture contains a mixture of four important species:

1. Intracellular $^{14}$C-thymine
2. Intracellular radiolabeled DNA
3. Extracellular $^{14}$C-thymine: unincorporated and from lysed cells
4. Extracellular radiolabeled DNA: from lysed cells only

We are only interested in quantifying the amount of radiolabel incorporated into DNA over the entire course of this experiment. Doing so would require us to assay DNA from existing cells (**intracellular DNA**) and lysed cells (**extracellular DNA**).

Likewise, we are not interested in assaying any $^{14}$C-thymine.

Simply **centrifuging** the cells and assaying the pellet would cause us to neglect extracellular DNA while also assaying unwanted intracellular $^{14}$C-thymine.

**Trichloroacetic acid** precipitation allows us to **isolate all DNA** while **ignoring $^{14}$C-thymine**.

Figure 6.3 shows that **nalidixic acid completely inhibits DNA replication**. For DNA, $^{14}$C-thymine incorporation is completely halted in the nalidixic acid-treated condition versus untreated control.

**Nalidixic acid does not significantly inhibit RNA or protein synthesis**. For both protein and RNA, there is a negligible but observable decrease in the incorporation of their radiolabeled precursors ($^{14}$C-L-arginine and $^{14}$C-uracil, respectively) in the nalidixic acid-treated condition versus untreated control. This slight decrease in incorporation/synthesis can be attributed to the **downchain effects** of the inhibition of DNA replication.

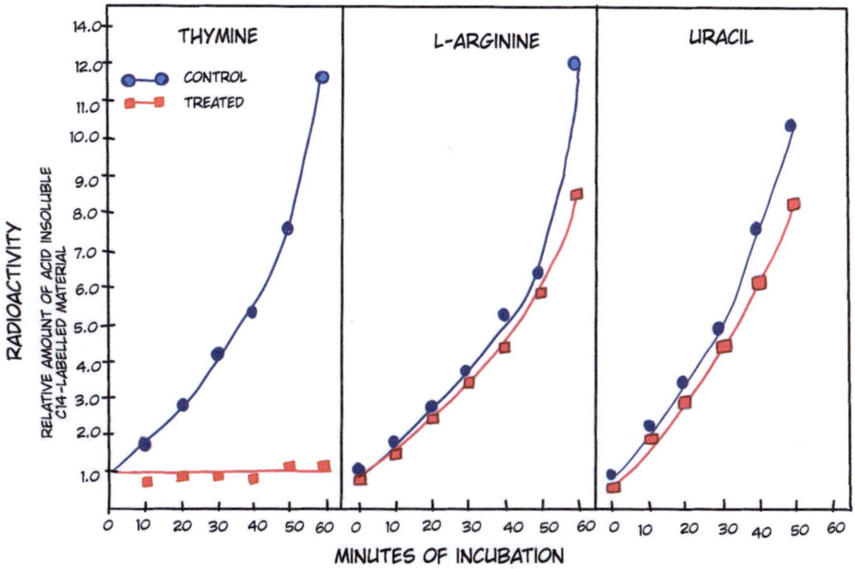


**Fig. 6.3** **Radioassay** to track the **synthesis of DNA, protein, and RNA** using their respective $^{14}$**C-labeled** substrates: **thymine, L-arginine**, and u**racil**. The addition of nalidixic acid appears to greatly **inhibit thymine utilization** (DNA replication) compared to L-arginine or uracil utilization (protein and RNA synthesis, respectively) [4]

► **Remark**

Gyrase removes two positive supercoils on DNA *in vivo*. It does this by **introducing two negative supercoils** into the strand. However, gyrase can introduce negative supercoils into any form of DNA, even relaxed DNA. This means that gyrase can still **supercoil a relaxed plasmid** *in vitro* by **introducing negative supercoils**. It should be noted that gyrase removes positive supercoils far faster than it can introduce negative supercoils [5].

## 6.4.1 Inhibition of Gyrase

**Agarose gel electrophoresis** is used to detect gyrase inhibition based on the principle that **supercoiled DNA travels faster** along the gel than uncoiled DNA [6].

Untreated relaxed plasmid will run a short distance through an agarose gel (Fig. 6.4, lane 1).

The activity of gyrase alone is tested by incubating the enzyme with relaxed plasmid and running it on an agarose gel. Gyrase is expected to negatively supercoil the plasmid, and any supercoiled form is expected to run faster than the relaxed form. A far greater amount of supercoiled form, and a far lesser amount of relaxed form, therefore indicates greater gyrase activity (Fig. 6.4, lane 2).

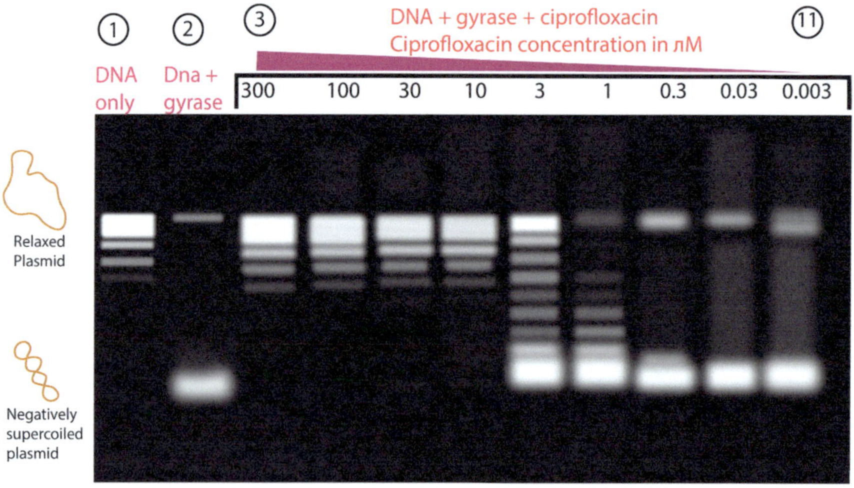


**Fig. 6.4** Agarose gel electrophoresis helps determine whether ciprofloxacin inhibits gyrase [6] (artist's impression). **Lane 1:** Untreated, **relaxed plasmid** showing a band that travels a shorter distance through the gel. **Lane 2:** Relaxed plasmid **treated with gyrase**, thereby producing a **negatively supercoiled** form showing a band that travels a longer distance through the gel. **Lanes 11 → 3:** Relaxed plasmid + gyrase + **ciprofloxacin**. At low concentrations of ciprofloxacin (lane 11), negatively supercoiled plasmid still dominates. This reverses at high concentrations (lane 3), when relaxed plasmid dominates. These results together confirm gyrase inhibition by ciprofloxacin

Quinolones (like ciprofloxacin) are expected to inhibit gyrase activity. Therefore, when introduced into a solution containing relaxed plasmid and gyrase, the opposite of lane 2 is observed: more of the relaxed form and less of the supercoiled form. This effect should be **concentration dependent** (Fig. 6.4, lanes 11 → 3).

### Technique 6.1

**Agarose gel electrophoresis** can be used to separate and visualize DNA based on differences in length and supercoiled state.

Agarose is highly purified agar that is stripped of all its impurities and possesses a neutral charge. Just like agar, it can be set as a gel. While setting the gel, *wells* or small, deep holes can also be created by placing a *comb* at the desired position before the gel sets. After the gel is cast, DNA is pipetted into these wells. The DNA is mixed with glycerol to ensure it sinks to the bottom of the well and with a purple dye (bromophenol) to track its initial location. Note that bromophenol does not stain the DNA itself, but ethidium bromide does. When placed within an electric field, negatively charged DNA will travel toward the positively charged cathode. DNA can then be visualized under UV light.

The distance traveled by DNA on an agarose gel depends on two factors:

1. **Length**: Longer molecules travel slower as they will continuously get entangled with the agarose substrate.
2. **Supercoiled state**: Highly supercoiled circular DNA will travel faster than relaxed circular DNA molecules of the same length. Supercoiled DNA will be able to pass through pores in the agarose substrate easier than relaxed DNA.

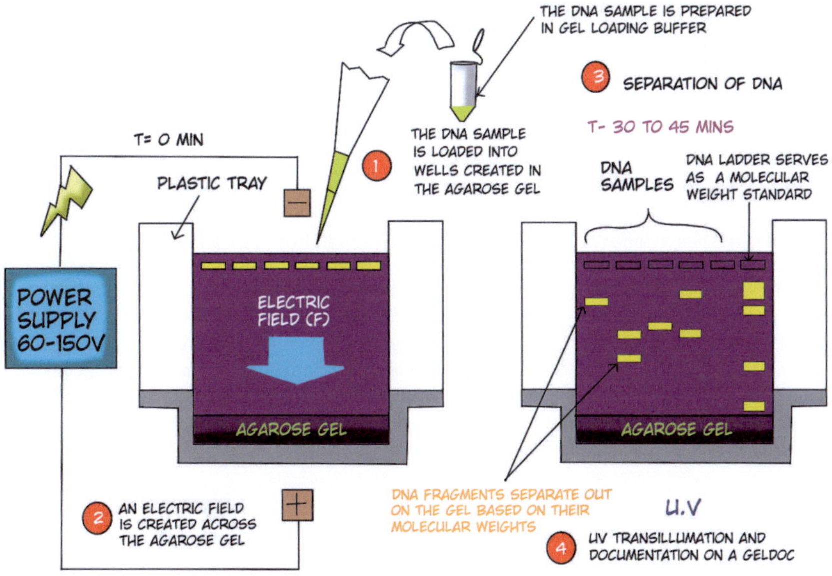

### 6.4.2 Crystal Structure

X-ray crystallography for crystals of gyrase bound to quinolones has been performed for a multitude of drugs and species. We will use a moxifloxacin/*Mycobacterium tuberculosis* gyrase crystal as a representative structure [7] (Fig. 6.5).

Despite their small size, quinolones interact with both the DNA double helix and the gyrase protein subunits. Quinolones accomplish this through two separate methods:

1. $\pi - \pi$ **stacking** interactions to intercalate with DNA, in a manner similar to DNA base stacking
2. Coordinate bonds linking moxifloxacin to a **magnesium atom**, which in turn interacts with protein residues through hydrogen bonded **water molecules**

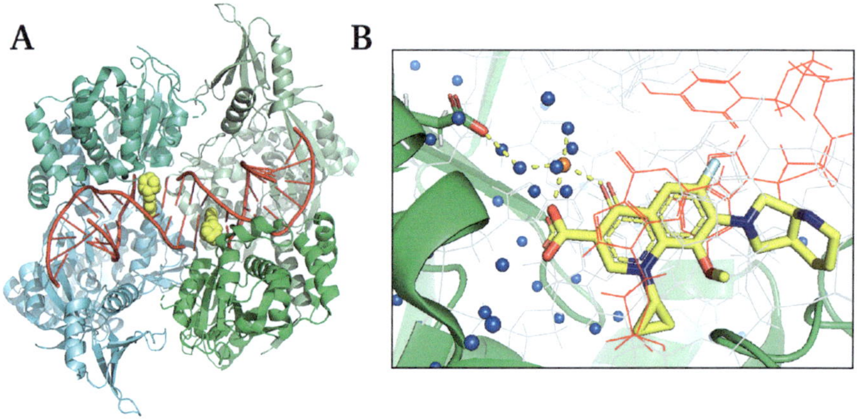


**Fig. 6.5 X-ray crystal structure of moxifloxacin bound to *M. tuberculosis* gyrase**. PDB ID: 5bs8 [7]. **(a) Overview** of the gyrase protein bound to moxifloxacin. Four protein chains are colored in different shades of blue/green. The DNA double helix is colored red. Moxifloxacin is colored yellow. **(b) Binding site** of moxifloxacin. The protein backbone is colored green. DNA is colored gray if not interacting with moxifloxacin and red if there are interactions. Moxifloxacin and the purine base immediately above it (in red) are on parallel planes, indicating a $\pi - \pi$ stacking interaction. The magnesium atom is colored orange and shown as a sphere. Oxygen atoms from water molecules are colored blue and shown as spheres. The intricate coordinate/hydrogen bonding network that connects moxifloxacin to the protein chain via magnesium and oxygen is shown as yellow dotted lines. Oxygen atoms (hydrogen bond acceptors) are colored red. Nitrogen atoms (hydrogen bond donors) are colored blue

## 6.5 Quinolone Resistance Mechanisms

Quinolone resistance mechanism can broadly be divided into two categories [8]:

1. **Mutations** to the quinolone binding site on **gyrase**, more common in gram-negative bacteria. Mutations may arise on either the GyrA or GyrB subunits. On the GyrA subunit, mutations tend to cluster on the quinolone resistance-determining region (QRDR). The QRDR represents the portion of GyrA protein that binds to DNA. **Topoisomerase IV** mutations (an alternate quinolone target) are more common in gram-positive bacteria.
2. **Efflux pumps** to remove the quinolone drug from the cytoplasm and eject it into the extracellular media. Read Sect. 3.4.3 for more details.

## 6.6 Problems

**Problem 6.1**

Can short (approx. 10,000 base pairs) linear supercoiled DNA exist in solution? Can a linear eukaryotic chromosome (approx. 60 million base pairs) exist in solution as supercoiled DNA? Explain for both.

**Problem 6.2**

You are attempting to perform a radioassay on a new quinolone antibiotic to check for inhibition of DNA replication exactly as described in the text. You check your stocks, and you have ample $^{14}C$-labeled L-arginine and uracil. However, you are out of radiolabeled thymine.
A project assistant working under you suggests using your stock of $^{32}PO_4^{3-}$ instead. She argues that $^{32}P$ will be incorporated into DNA as part of the phosphate backbone.
Do you listen to your project assistant's advice? Why or why not?

**Problem 6.3**

Design an experiment to differentiate between positively supercoiled and negatively supercoiled plasmid. Assume both plasmids have the same number of supercoils.

**Problem 6.4**

Your guide has synthesized a new quinolone antibiotic that he expects to inhibit gyrase. He asks you to use the standard agarose gel electrophoresis technique to test its efficacy. When going through your reagents, you realize that you have everything you need except for relaxed plasmid. However, you have a large stock of positively supercoiled plasmid at hand.

Design an experiment that uses positively supercoiled plasmid instead of relaxed plasmid. Draw your expected results.

**Problem 6.5**

A new bacterial gyrase (Ngyr) is discovered that may induce either positive or negative supercoils on a given plasmid. Design an experiment to determine which the case is. Draw a diagram containing your expected observations.

**Problem 6.6**

Quinones interact with gyrase via $\pi$-$\pi$ stacking interactions. You have observed this in the X-ray crystal structure of the complex (Fig. 6.5). Design another experiment to confirm this is the case.

## References


1. Bisacchi GS (2015) Origins of the quinolone class of antibacterials: an expanded "discovery story" miniperspective. J Med Chem 58(12):4874–4882
2. King DE, Malone R, Lilley SH (2000) New classification and update on the quinolone antibiotics. Am Family Physician 61(9):2741–2748
3. Vos SM, Tretter EM, Schmidt BH, Berger JM (2011) All tangled up: how cells direct, manage and exploit topoisomerase function. Nature Rev Mol Cell Biol 12(12):827–841
4. Goss WA, Deitz WH, Cook TM (1965) Mechanism of action of nalidixic acid on *Escherichia coli* II. inhibition of deoxyribonucleic acid synthesis. J Bacteriol 89(4):1068–1074
5. Ashley RE, Dittmore A, McPherson SA, Turnbough CL Jr, Neuman KC, Osheroff N (2017) Activities of gyrase and topoisomerase iv on positively supercoiled DNA. Nucl Acids Res 45(16):9611–9624
6. Mitchenall LA, Hipkin RE, Piperakis MM, Burton NP, Maxwell A (2018) A rapid high-resolution method for resolving DNA topoisomers. BMC Res Notes 11(1):1–7
7. Blower TR, Williamson BH, Kerns RJ, Berger JM (2016) Crystal structure and stability of gyrase–fluoroquinolone cleaved complexes from *Mycobacterium tuberculosis*. Proc Natl Acad Sci 113(7):1706–1713
8. Blondeau JM (2004) Fluoroquinolones: mechanism of action, classification, and development of resistance. Survey Pphthalmol 49(2):S73–S78

# Rifampicin

# 7

Deepesh Nagarajan

**Abstract**

Rifampicin is an antibiotic used to treat tuberculosis. It was discovered by Hermes Pagani from a soil actinomycete. Rifampicin inhibits transcription. Rifampicin binds to the $\beta$ subunit deep within the DNA/RNA channel of bacterial RNA polymerase, thereby directly blocking the elongation of RNA. Rifampicin binding to RNA polymerase can be confirmed by intrinsic fluorescence quenching experiments. Rifampicin causes abortive initiation or the release of short RNA fragments rather than full m-RNA transcripts. Radiolabeled abortive initiation transcripts are detectable on a PAGE gel. The X-ray crystal structure of the rifampicin-RNA polymerase complex confirms that it binds to the $\beta$ subunit of *Thermus aquaticus* RNA polymerase. Mutations to the rpoG gene, which encodes the $\beta$ subunit, confer rifampicin resistance. Multidrug efflux pumps can also remove intracellular rifampicin.

**Keywords**

Quinolone · Gyrase · Supercoiling · Antibiotic resistance

Rifampicin (Fig. 7.1) is an antibiotic used to treat several types of bacterial infections, including tuberculosis, *Mycobacterium avium* complex, leprosy, and Legionnaires' disease. For treating tuberculosis, rifampicin is usually coadmin-

D. Nagarajan (✉)
Department of Biotechnology, M.S. Ramaiah University of Applied Sciences, Bangalore, India

Department of Microbiology, St. Xavier's College, Mumbai, India
e-mail: deepeshn.bt.ls@msruas.ac.in; deepesh.nagarajan@xaviers.edu

© The Editor(s) (if applicable) and The Author(s), under exclusive license to Springer Nature Singapore Pte Ltd. 2024

D. Nagarajan (ed.), *Antibiotics and Their Mechanisms of Action*,
https://doi.org/10.1007/978-981-97-6851-6_7

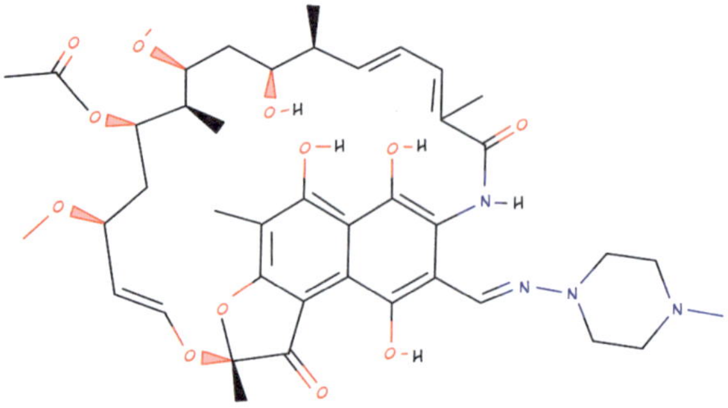

**Fig. 7.1** Structure of rifampicin

istered with other antituberculosis antibiotics like pyrazinamide, isoniazid, and ethambutol.

Rifampicin is administered either orally or intravenously. Common side effects include nausea, vomiting, diarrhea, and loss of appetite. Serious side effects include hepatotoxicity and allergic reactions. One unusual side effect is that it often turns urine, sweat, and tears a red or an orange color.

Rifampicin is produced by the soil bacterium *Amycolatopsis rifamycinica*, an **actinomycete**. It was discovered by **Hermes Pagani** in 1965. The antibiotic was named after "Rififi," the title of a popular movie at the time (Fig. 7.2). Rifampicin was further developed in Dow-Lepetit Research Laboratories (Milan, Italy). It was marketed in Italy in 1967 and approved in the USA in 1971.

## 7.1 Transcription

Before dealing with rifampicin's mechanism of action, a recap of bacterial transcription (Fig. 7.3) is needed.

Bacterial transcription is the process in which a segment of bacterial DNA is copied into a newly synthesized strand of messenger RNA (mRNA) with the use of the enzyme **RNA polymerase** (Fig. 7.4). The process occurs in three main steps: **initiation**, **elongation**, and **termination**, and the end result is a strand of mRNA that is complementary to a single strand of DNA.

### 7.1.1 RNA Polymerase

In most prokaryotes, a single RNA polymerase species transcribes all types of RNA. The RNA polymerase "core" from *Escherichia coli* consists of five subunits: $\alpha^{I}$, $\alpha^{II}$, $\beta$, $\beta'$,, and $\omega$.

The $\beta$ **subunits** are most important. They contain the active center responsible for **RNA synthesis**, as well as residues that nonspecifically interact with DNA and newly formed RNA.

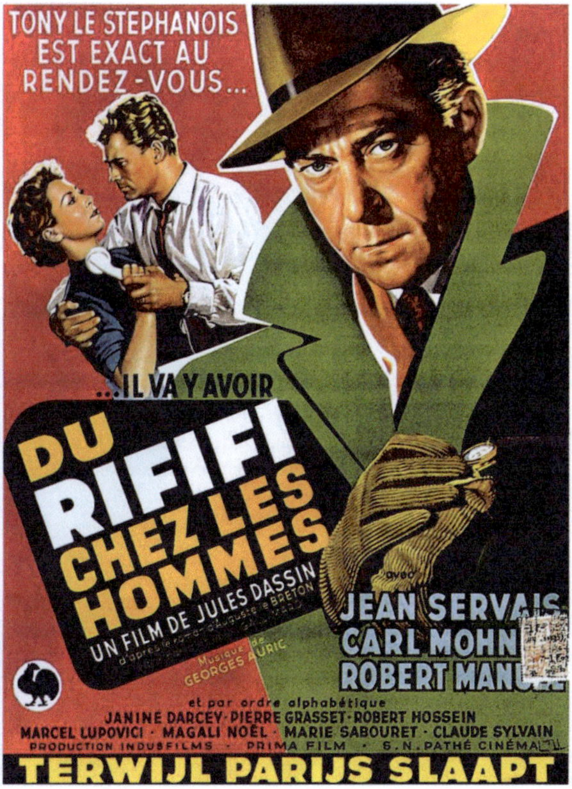


**Fig. 7.2** Poster for "Rififi," a 1955 French noir/crime film that lent its name to rifampicin

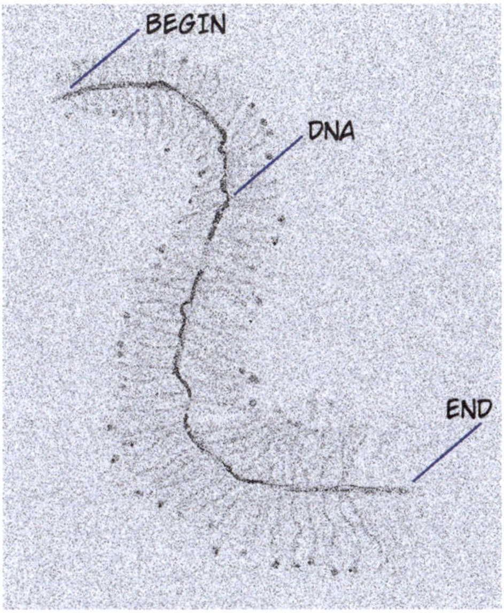


**Fig. 7.3** **Electron microscopic image of RNA transcription**. The forming RNA strands are visible as branches from the main DNA strand. Transcription was occurring from right to left. RNA transcripts get longer as the RNA polymerases progress down the gene (artist's impression)

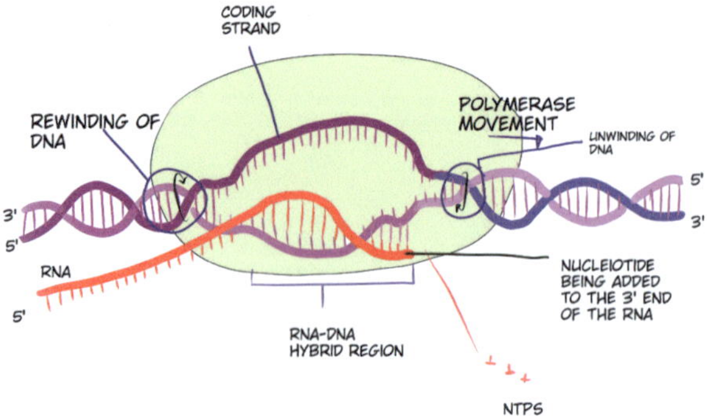


**Fig. 7.4** A representation of **RNA polymerase** during the elongation phase of RNA synthesis. RNA polymerase moves along the coding strand of DNA in a 3'→5' direction. Single nucleoside triphosphates (NTPs) are polymerized into an RNA strand that is synthesized in the 5'→3' direction. Positive supercoils are generated ahead of RNA polymerase. Negative supercoils are generated behind the complex

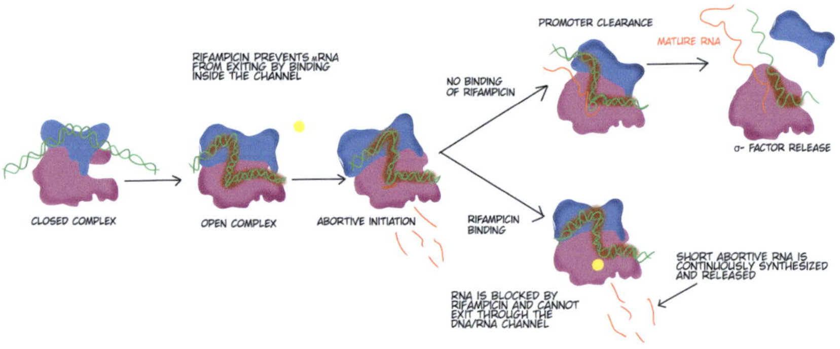


**Fig. 7.5** Steps involved in **transcription initiation**. Transcription proceeds normally and culminates in the release of mature mRNA without rifampicin. If rifampicin is introduced, transcription stalls at abortive initiation indefinitely

A small **sigma** (*σ*) **factor** also binds to this core to initiate transcription. After transcription starts, the factor can unbind and let the core enzyme proceed with its work. The core RNA polymerase complex forms a **crab claw** or **clamp-jaw** structure with an internal channel running along the full length.

### 7.1.2 Transcription Initiation

Understanding transcription initiation [1] (Fig. 7.5) is a prerequisite for understanding rifampicin's mechanism of action.

Initiation begins when bacterial *σ* **factors** guide and position the RNA polymerase complex, causing it to bind to promoters on the DNA double helix. Most genes are transcribed with the help of the housekeeping $\sigma$ factor, although alternate $\sigma$ factors exist for some genes.

Once bound, RNA polymerase transitions from a **closed complex** to an **open complex** by unwinding the DNA double helix in the region of the transcription start site. $\sigma$ factors also help orchestrate the formation of the open complex.

The open complex transitions into the **initiation complex** with the addition of nucleoside triphosphates (NTPs) and begins to synthesize the RNA transcript.

Initially, **scrunching** occurs. Here, the unwound DNA double helix is pulled into the initiating complex and forms small single-stranded loops. This causes the RNA polymerase to initially stall at the promoter. This results in cycles of **abortive initiation** that produce **short RNA strands** varying in length from 2 to 10 nucleotides and are highly dependent on their parent exons. Eventually, the RNA polymerase escapes the promoter, releases the $\sigma$ factor, and enters the **elongation phase**.

## 7.2 Mechanism of Action

Rifampin binds to and **inhibits bacterial RNA polymerase**. The drug binds to the $\beta$ subunit deep within the DNA/RNA channel, thereby directly **blocking the elongation of RNA** (Fig. 7.5).

### 7.2.1 Binding to RNA Polymerase

Rifampicin binding to the core RNA polymerase (excluding $\sigma$ factor) of *E. coli* was confirmed by exploiting rifampicin's ability to **quench (decrease) the intrinsic fluorescence** of proteins.

When excited at 290 nm, proteins fluoresce at 335 nm. Rifampicin bound to any protein, including RNA polymerase, will quench this intrinsic fluorescence. The amount of rifampicin bound to RNA polymerase can therefore be estimated by measuring the decrease in protein fluorescence from its unbound peak. Fluorescence quenching experiments confirmed that rifampicin binds to RNA polymerase (Fig. 7.6a).

By observing the change in fluorescence upon adding small amounts of rifampicin to RNA polymerase and by noting the point at which the fluorescence no longer changes, it is also possible to perform a titration experiment. Such an experiment revealed that rifampicin bound to RNA polymerase with a **1:1 stoichiometric ratio** (Fig. 7.6b).

It should be noted that Rifampicin is an exception in this regard, as most drugs do not cause intrinsic fluorescence quenching in proteins.

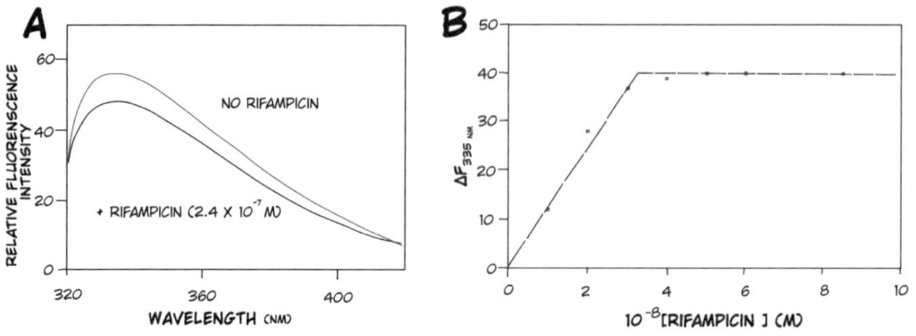


**Fig. 7.6** **Intrinsic fluorescence quenching** confirms rifampicin-RNA polymerase binding. **(a)** Change in intrinsic fluorescence of *E. coli* RNA polymerase. Free RNA polymerase shows a relative fluorescence intensity of approximately 60 units at 335 nm. RNA polymerase bound to rifampicin shows a decreased fluorescence intensity of $\leq$50 units at 335 nm. **(b)** Titration experiment using the aforementioned decrease in fluorescence to obtain the stoichiometric ratio, which was determined to be 1:1. Excitation: 290 nm/emission: 335 nm for both panels

### 7.2.2 Inhibition of RNA Elongation

Rifampicin does not interfere with the binding of bacterial RNA polymerase to DNA and transcription initiation. However, rifampicin blocks the elongation of RNA and the release of mature mRNA.

This can be demonstrated by an experiment that tracks the release of short nascent radiolabeled RNA molecules during **abortive initiation** [2].

A cell-free reaction mix containing *E. coli* RNA polymerase, DNA from bacteriophage T7, and all nucleotide triphosphates for RNA synthesis (ATP, GTP, CTP, and [$^{32}$P]UTP) was prepared for this experiment. The A1 promoter was chosen as the transcription site. To ensure its sole transcription, promoters A2 and A3 were deleted. A 5'-**CpA**-3' primer was added as an artificial transcription initiator.

Three transcription products were observed:

1. **Radiolabeled CpApU** abortive initiation products, whose concentration increased with an increasing concentration of rifampicin. This confirms the inhibition of RNA elongation by the drug.
2. A 105 nucleotide **terminated transcript**. Its concentration decreased with increasing rifampicin.
3. A 127 nucleotide **runoff transcript** that overshot the tR2 intrinsic terminator. Its concentration also decreased with increasing rifampicin.

These products were observed after running radioactive reaction mixtures on a 15% acrylamide gel (which can also be used for nucleic acids), collecting autoradiographs, and noting band patterns and intensities (Fig. 7.7).

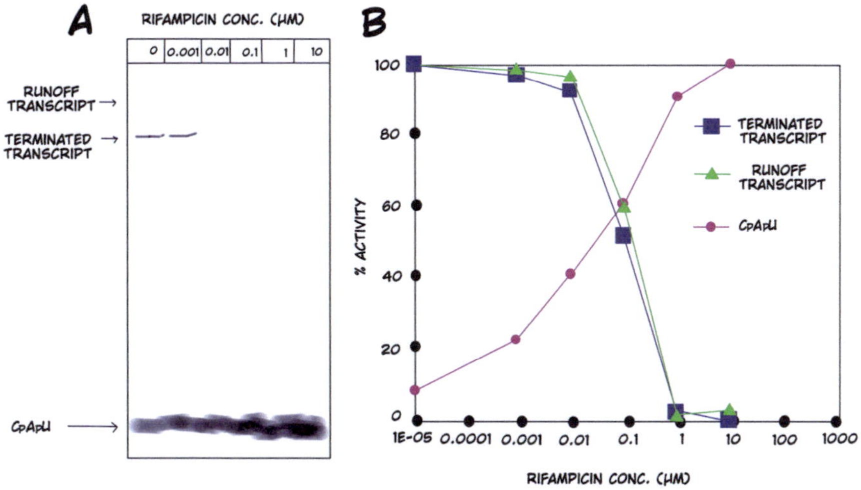


**Fig. 7.7** **Radioassay that demonstrates rifampicin's mechanism of action** [2]. **(a)** Increase in CpApu concentration and decrease in terminated/runoff transcript with increasing rifampicin concentration (artist's impression). Cell-free reaction mixtures were prepared as described in the text and only differed in the concentration of rifampicin. These mixtures were run on a 15% polyacrylamide gel to separate the transcripts based on length. **(b)** Quantitative plot expressing radiation intensity from the autoradiograph in **(a)** as percentage activity

These three observations confirm that:

1. **Rifampicin does not interfere with RNA polymerase/DNA binding**. If that were the case, then abortive transcripts could not have been transcribed.
2. **Rifampicin prevents transcription elongation**. The concentration of CpApU increases, and the concentrations of the terminated and runoff transcript decrease, with increasing concentrations of rifampicin.

### 7.2.3 Crystal Structure

X-ray crystallography was used to solve the rifampicin-bound structure of *Thermus aquaticus* RNA polymerase [3]. This protein was used as a model for all other bacterial RNA polymerases due to its amenability to crystallization.

The structure confirmed that rifampicin binds to a pocket within the $\beta$ subunit of *T. aquaticus* RNA polymerase (Fig. 7.8). Unlike fluoroquinolones (see Sect. 6.4.2), rifampicin does not directly interact with any nucleic acids. Instead, the presence of rifampicin causes a steric hindrance in the DNA/RNA channel that prevents newly synthesized mRNA from exiting.

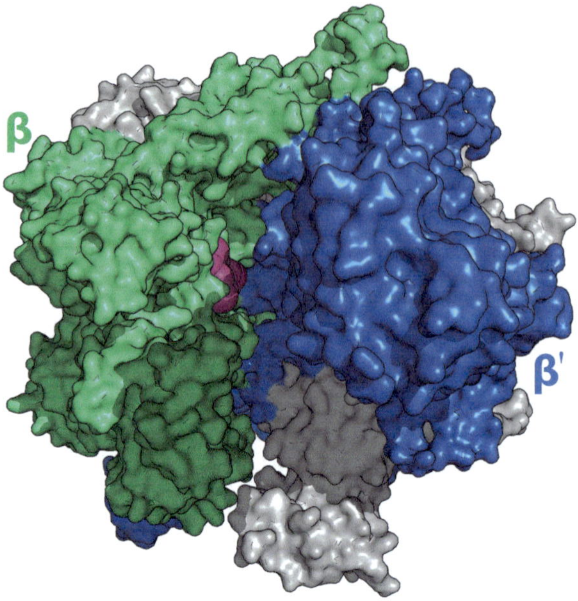


**Fig. 7.8 Crystal structure of *T. aquaticus* RNA polymerase bound to rifampicin.** PDB ID: 1ynn [3]. Rifampicin is colored magenta. The $\beta$ subunit is colored green. The $\beta$' subunit is colored blue. Together the $\beta\beta$' subunits form the DNA/RNA channel

## 7.3 Rifampicin Resistance Mechanisms

Bacteria can evolve rifampicin resistance through two main mechanisms:

1. **Mutations to the rpoB gene**, which encodes the RNA polymerase $\beta$ subunit [4]. These mutations occur at the rifampicin binding site and decrease protein–drug binding affinity.
2. **Efflux pumps** that remove intracellular rifampicin and eject it into the extracellular media. Read Sect. 3.4.3 for more details.

## 7.4 Problems

**Problem 7.1**

Assume that rifampicin did not cause intrinsic fluorescence quenching in proteins. Design another experiment to detect rifampicin/RNA polymerase binding.

**Problem 7.2**

How would you use the radioassay depicted in Fig. 6.3 to confirm rifampicin's mechanism of action? Draw your expected results.

**Problem 7.3**

A new RNA polymerase inhibitor is suspected to act by inhibiting transcription termination, rather than transcription initiation. Design an experiment to confirm that this is the case.

**Problem 7.4**

Why do quinolones inhibit DNA synthesis but not transcription? Both processes involve the unwinding and rewinding of DNA.

## References

1. Browning DF, Busby SJW (2016) Local and global regulation of transcription initiation in bacteria. Nature Rev Microbiol 14(10):638–650
2. Campbell EA, Korzheva N, Mustaev A, Murakami K, Nair S, Goldfarb A, Darst SA (2001) Structural mechanism for rifampicin inhibition of bacterial RNA polymerase. Cell 104(6):901–912
3. Campbell EA, Pavlova O, Zenkin N, Leon F, Irschik H, Jansen R, Severinov K, Darst SA (2005) Structural, functional, and genetic analysis of sorangicin inhibition of bacterial RNA polymerase. EMBO J 24(4):674–682
4. Cai X-C, Xi H, Liang L, Liu J-D, Liu C-H, Xue Y-R, Yu X-Y (2017) Rifampicin-resistance mutations in the rpoB gene in *Bacillus velezensis* cc09 have pleiotropic effects. Front Microbiol 8:178

# Tetracyclines

# 8

Deepesh Nagarajan

**Abstract**

Tetracyclines are a group of broad spectrum antibiotics that all share a common naphthacene core structure. Tetracyclines are named after the eponymous tetracycline, which was a first generation drug of this class. Second and third generation drugs such as doxycycline, minocycline, tigecycline, and eravacycline are also in clinical use. Tetracycline binds to the A-site of the bacterial ribosome found within the 30S subunit, preventing aminoacyl tRNA from attaching, thereby inhibiting translation. The molecular mechanism of action of tetracycline is complicated. A large number of experiments performed by different groups over a period of decades was required to decipher this mechanism of action. These experiments relied heavily on cell-free ribosomal reaction mixtures capable if in vitro translation. Other experiments involved radioassays using $^3$H-labelled tetracycline, sucrose density gradient centrifugation of whole ribosomes and ribosomal subunits, 2D urea PAGE electrophoresis of photoincorporated tetracycline, and X-ray crystallography. It should be noted that this consensus has been challenged in recent years. Tetracycline resistance can arise through mutations in 16S rRNA, the evolution of tetracycline-hydroxylating enzymes, ribosomal protection proteins, and through the use of multidrug efflux pumps.

**Keywords**

Tetracycline · Sucrose density gradient centrifugation · 2D PAGE · Photolabelling · Antibiotic resistance

D. Nagarajan (✉)
Department of Biotechnology, M.S. Ramaiah University of Applied Sciences, Bangalore, India

Department of Microbiology, St. Xavier's College, Mumbai, India
e-mail: deepeshn.bt.ls@msruas.ac.in; deepesh.nagarajan@xaviers.edu

© The Editor(s) (if applicable) and The Author(s), under exclusive license to Springer Nature Singapore Pte Ltd. 2024

D. Nagarajan (ed.), *Antibiotics and Their Mechanisms of Action*, https://doi.org/10.1007/978-981-97-6851-6_8

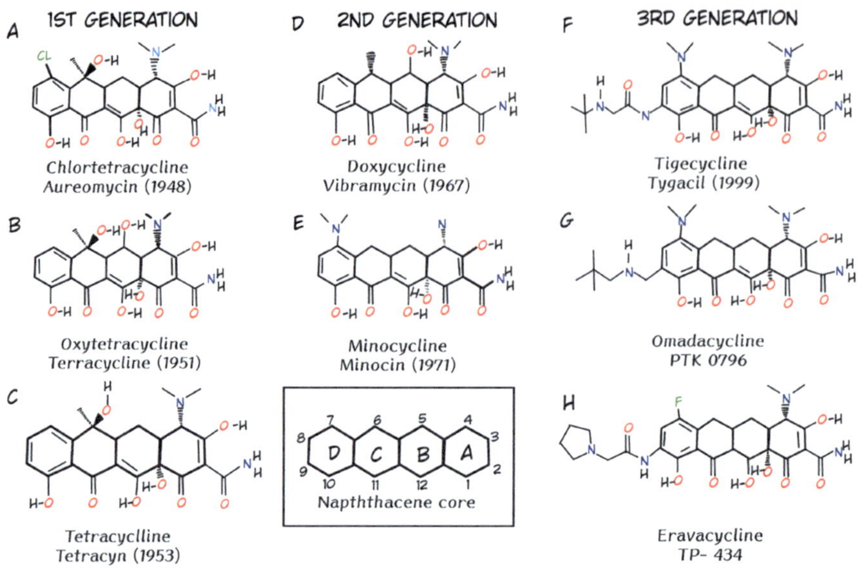


**Fig. 8.1** **Structures of important tetracycline drugs**. Year of discovery also indicated in brackets. Tetracyclines of the **first generation**. (**a**) Chlortetracycline, (**b**) oxytetracycline, (**c**) tetracycline. Tetracyclines of the **second generation**: (**d**) doxycycline, (**e**) minocycline. Tetracyclines of the **third generation**: (**f**) tigecycline, (**g**) omadacycline, (**h**) eravacycline. Inset: carbon atom assignments within the naphthacene core

Tetracyclines are a group of broad spectrum, bacteriostatic antibiotics used to treat diseases ranging from acne to anthrax. All tetracyclines share a common naphthacene core structure (Fig. 8.1). Various side chains attached to this naphthacene core contribute to the tetracycline family's varying functional properties.

## 8.1 The Ribosome as a Drug Target

At least seven antibiotic classes inhibit the bacterial ribosome (Fig. 8.2). This constitutes a number greater than for any other antibacterial drug target discovered to date:

1. **Tetracyclines** bind to the aminoacyl site (A-site) and prevent aminoacyl-tRNA from entering. This prevents the elongation of the nascent polypeptide chain.
2. **Aminoglycosides** (e.g., streptomycin, gentamycin, amikacin) cause codon misreading. The translated polypeptide chains will possess a sequence very different from that encoded in its mRNA.
3. **Lincosamides** (e.g., clindamycin) inhibit peptidyl transferase activity, preventing the peptide bond from forming.
4. **Streptogramins** (e.g., virginiamycin) also inhibit peptidyl transferase activity.

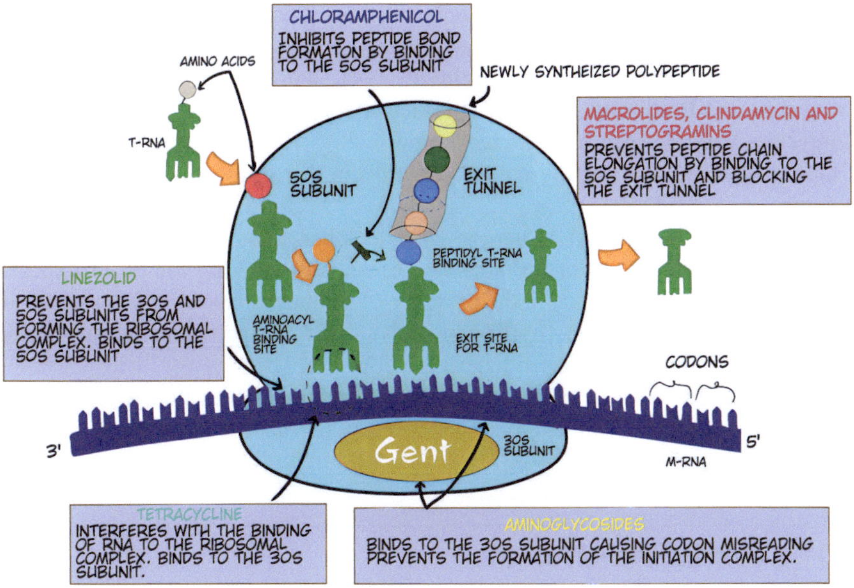


**Fig. 8.2** **Antibiotics that target the ribosome** along with their specific targets

5. **Chloramphenicol** also inhibits peptidyl transferase activity.
6. **Macrolides** (e.g., erythromycin, azithromycin, clarithromycin) bind to the exit tunnel and prevent the nascent polypeptide chain from exiting.
7. **Oxazolidinones** (e.g., linezolid) prevent the 30S and 50S ribosomal subunits from assembling.

Protein synthesis is absolutely essential to the survival of a pathogen and is performed by a **single protein complex**. Inhibiting the ribosome can therefore bring all cellular processes to a halt. While this makes the ribosome an appealing drug target, it still does not explain the ribosome's disproportionate targeting.

Protein synthesis is a multistep biochemical reaction. Ribosomal recognition of mRNA, ribosomal assembly, peptidyl-tRNA binding to the A-site, peptide bond formation, ribosomal translocation, nascent protein escape from the E-site, nascent polypeptide escape through the polypeptide exit tunnel, and ribosomal disassembly are all distinct processes that can be targeted by distinct antibiotics. In effect, the ribosome constitutes a **dozen drug targets bundled into a single protein complex**.

## 8.2 History

Tetracycline consumption can be traced to antiquity with the discovery of fluorescently labelled bones from Nubian mummies dated between 350 and 550 A.D. [1]. Tetracycline is fluorescent and has a strong affinity for calcium, including hydroxyapatite found in bones. The source of this tetracycline is unknown but may have come from beer brewed from contaminated grain [2].

Tetracycline's modern history begins in 1948, with the discovery of **chlortetracycline** by **Benjamin Duggar**. Chlortetracycline was isolated from the actinomycete *Streptomyces aureofaciens* (now called *Kitasatospora aureofaciens*). Chlortetracycline was initially named aureomycin due to the golden coloration of colonies of its producer.

Aureomycin's chemical structure was deciphered in 1952, which enabled researchers to try and rationally alter it. Researchers working for Pfizer exposed chlortetracycline to hydrogen in the presence of a catalyst, causing the replacement of chlorine with hydrogen (**hydrogenolysis**). This new compound was named **tetracycline** and displayed considerably superior properties.

Further tetracyclines belonging to the second and third generations were likewise created through the chemical functionalization of the natural chlortetracycline molecule (Fig. 8.1).

## 8.3 Mechanism of Action

1. Tetracycline binds to the ribosome.
2. Nonspecific, reversible tetracycline:ribosome binding is observable at stoichiometric ratios as high as 100:1.
3. Specific, irreversible tetracycline:ribosome binding occurs in a 1:1 stoichiometric ratio.
4. Tetracycline inhibits protein synthesis.
5. Tetracycline prevents aminoacyl tRNA from attaching to the aminoacyl site (A-site).
6. The current academic consensus is that tetracycline targets the 30S ribosomal subunit, although this consensus has been challenged.

Each of the above steps can be experimentally verified and will be discussed in detail below.

**Remark**

A fair understanding of protein translation is a prerequisite to understanding tetracycline's mechanism of action. You are encouraged to watch translation videos on youtube before reading this section. Examples:
https://youtu.be/Ikq9AcBcohA
https://youtu.be/KZBljAM6B1s
https://youtu.be/7cn10wayDug

### 8.3.1 Ribosome Binding

Tetracycline binds to the bacterial ribosome. Recall that ligands that bind to a protein stabilize the protein in the process, as seen for the sypro orange thermal shift assay (Sect. 3.3.2). The use of sypro orange for tetracyclines is unnecessary as rRNA provides a comparable signal during thermal denaturation. **rRNA within the ribosome absorbs light at 260 nm**. Its absorbance decreases when bound to protein and increases when free. An increase in absorbance at 260 nm is therefore proportional to the amount of denatured ribosome.

An experiment using untreated and minocycline-treated ribosomes showed an increase in thermal stability upon minocycline treatment using this method, thereby indicating ribosome-tetracycline binding [3] (Fig. 8.3, Table 8.1).

### 8.3.2 Nonspecific Binding

Tetracycline is capable of binding to the ribosome in a weak, nonspecific, and easily reversible manner [4]. Several hundred tetracycline molecules can bind to a single ribosome in this binding mode. Total tetracycline binding can easily be assayed spectroscopically since **tetracycline absorbs light at 275 nm and 300 nm**. Such experiments confirmed that the vast majority of tetracycline bound to the ribosome does so weakly and can easily be sheared off by vigorous resuspension (protocol in Fig. 8.4, results in Fig. 8.5).

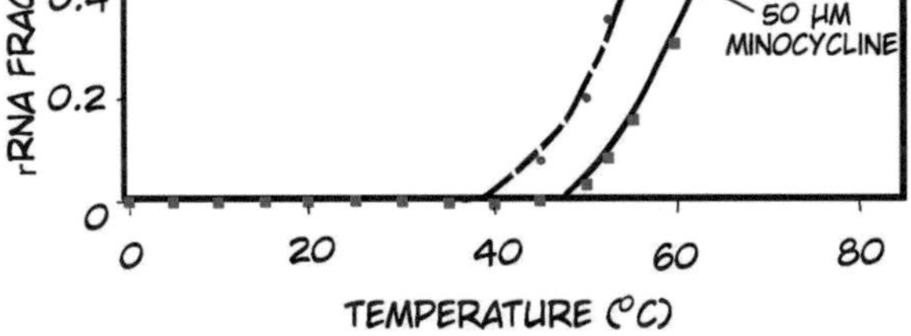


**Fig. 8.3 Tetracycline-ribosome binding** assayed using a thermal shift assay [3]. $T_m$ represents the temperature (in °C) at which half the ribosomes in solution have unfolded. Greater $T_m$ values indicate greater stabilization of the ribosome via tetracycline binding. Minocycline-bound ribosome possessed a $T_m$ of 68°C, which was 6.5°C higher than untreated ribosome

**Table 8.1** **Inhibition of protein synthesis by tetracycline** and its derivatives [3]. $T_m$ represents the temperature (in $°C$) at which half the ribosomes in solution have unfolded. Greater $T_m$ values indicate greater stabilization of the ribosome via tetracycline binding. $ID_{50}$ represents the concentration of tetracycline (in μM) required for half-maximal inhibition of $^{14}$C-polyphenylalanine synthesis. Lower concentrations indicate stronger ribosomal inhibition for a given antibiotic

| Tetracycline derivative | $T_m$ (°C) | $ID_{50}$ (μM) |
|---|---|---|
| Tetracycline | 62 | 14.8 |
| Oxytetracycline | 63 | 12 |
| Demethylchlortetracycline | 68 | 6.8 |
| Chlortetracycline | 64 | 5.8 |
| Methacycline | 66 | 4.8 |
| Minocycline | 68 | 3.2 |
| No drug (control) | 61.5 | N/A |

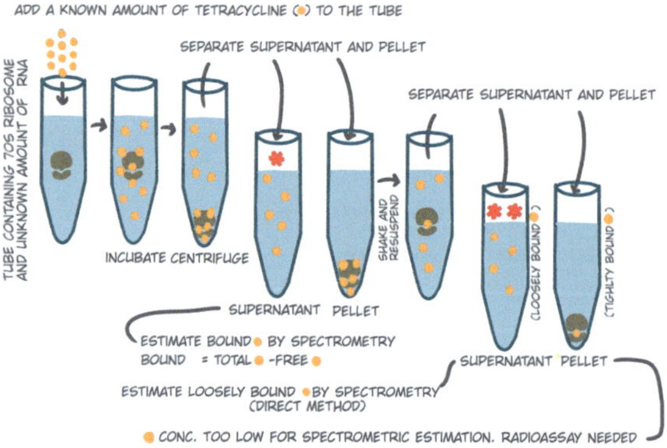


**Fig. 8.4** Protocol for assaying **nonspecific tetracycline binding** using spectroscopy [4]. *: Binding assay that measures all tetracycline bound to the ribosome. **: Nonspecific binding assay that measures the amount of tetracycline nonspecifically bound to the ribosome. Nonspecifically bound tetracycline should readily release from the ribosome pellet when vigorously resuspended. This assay cannot be used to estimate specifically bound tetracycline because spectroscopic assays are not sensitive enough to detect a 1:1 stoichiometry, and because some released tetracycline will rebind to the ribosome even after vigorous resuspension of the pellet

### 8.3.3 Specific Binding

Strong and irreversible binding occurs in an exact 1:1 ribosome:tetracycline stoichiometric ratio [4] (Fig. 8.6). Spectroscopic methods are not sensitive enough to quantify tetracycline at such low concentrations, and therefore a **radioassay** was used to calculate this ratio.

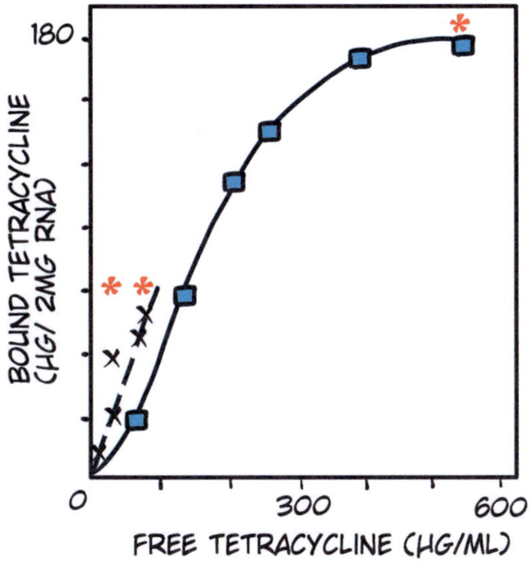


**Fig. 8.5 Nonspecific tetracycline binding** assayed using spectroscopy [4]. Various concentrations of tetracycline (x-axis) were incubated with ribosomes containing 2 mg of rRNA (see Fig. 8.4 for protocol for a single concentration of tetracycline). Solid line/*: All tetracycline bound to the ribosome. At the highest tetracycline concentration assayed, the mass ratio of bound tetracycline:rRNA was 180 µg:2 mg = 9:100, easily corresponding to several hundred tetracycline molecules per ribosome. Dotted line / **: Nonspecifically bound tetracycline. The amount of nonspecifically bound tetracycline was indistinguishable from the total amount of bound tetracycline (*). Note that due to the low sensitivity of this spectroscopic assay, the amount of nonspecifically bound tetracycline appears to be larger than the total amount of bound tetracycline, even though this is a logical impossibility

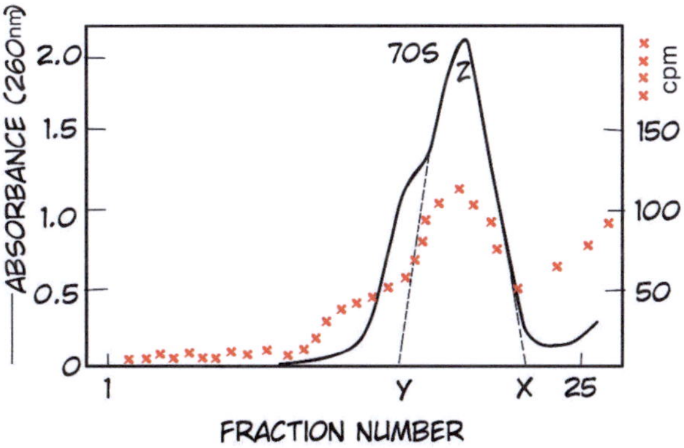


**Fig. 8.6 Radioassay to detect specific tetracycline:ribosome binding**, using a sucrose density gradient. cpm = counts per minute. Fractions y-x contain 70S ribosomes. z represents peak intensity/concentration

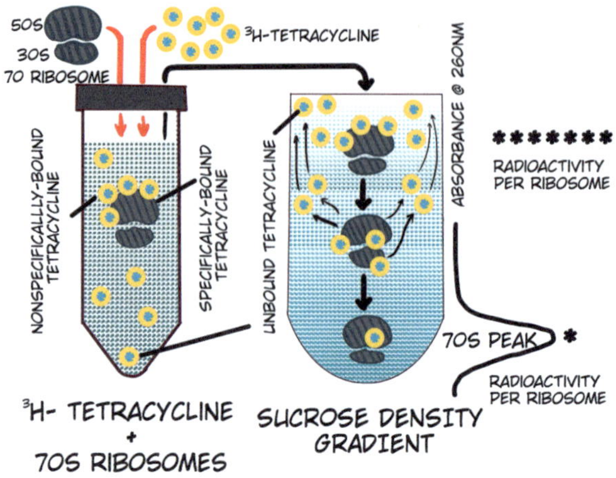


**Fig. 8.7** Protocol for measuring the stoichiometry of specifically bound $^{3}$H-tetracycline with the 70S ribosome

**70S ribosomes** were incubated with **$^{3}$H-labelled tetracycline** and subjected to centrifugation along a sucrose density gradient (Fig. 8.7). Centrifugation efficiently shears off all nonspecifically bound tetracycline, leaving only specifically bound tetracycline. After spinning, the column can be divided into fractions by pipetting out a predefined volume from the top of the tube.

For every fraction, ribosome concentration can be calculated from rRNA absorbance at 260 nm. Alternatively, some ultracentrifuges come equipped with inbuilt spectrophotometers that can analyze a centrifuge tube in situ.

Likewise, radiolabelled tetracycline concentration can be calculated from counts per minute (c.p.m) observed on a scintillation counter.

Using the summation of these two values across all fractions containing 70S ribosomes (y-x in Fig. 8.6), the ratio of specifically bound tetracycline:ribosome was found to be 1:1.

▶ **Remark**

Up to 40% of the ribosome's mass is composed of rRNA, allowing absorbance at 260 nm to be used to estimate ribosomal concentration. mRNA and tRNA interacting with the ribosome will only negligibly contribute to this signal.

## 8.3.4 Inhibition of Protein Synthesis

The effect of tetracycline on ribosomal function was studied using a cell-free extract capable of protein synthesis. The composition of this reaction mix and its preparation protocol are rather complex [5], but the main constituents are described below:

1. **70S ribosomes** obtained from sucrose density gradient centrifugation and stripped of their mRNA.
2. **Polyuracil (-(UUU)$_n$-)** which substitutes mRNA and codes for phenylalanine. Synthesizing a ribonucleic acid homopolymer is far easier than synthesizing a nonrandom heteropolymer that codes for a real protein. Polyuracil can also induce protein synthesis without the need for a start codon, with phe-tRNA directly binding to the P-site. However, polyphenylalanine synthesis from polyuracil occurs at a much slower rate compared to in vivo protein synthesis, polymerizing at a paltry rate of 280 residues hour$^{-1}$ ribosome$^{-1}$.
3. **Phenylalanyl-tRNA** extracted from a pellet of *E. coli* cells. The original method [6] for extraction was cumbersome and has been replaced by simpler affinity chromatography methods [7]. Using affinity chromatography, phenylalanyl-tRNAs can be pulled from an *E. coli* extract very simply using polyuracil (-(UUU)$_n$-) covalently linked to a column. The phenylalanyl group can be decoupled and replaced with radiolabelled phenylalanine for further experiments.
4. **ATP**, **GTP**, $Mg^{2+}$, EDTA, other small molecules, salts, and buffering compounds.

Naturally, this reaction mixture is expected to translate polyuracil into polyphenylalanine under baseline conditions in the absence of tetracycline (Fig. 8.8, untreated control). This can be assayed using $^{14}$C-phenylalanyl-tRNA and sucrose density gradient centrifugation (Fig. 8.9). Due to the slow rate of protein synthesis in the reaction mix, most polyphenylalanine will still be attached to the ribosome after 60 min. Polyphenylalanine concentration can then be quantified by observing radioactivity (counts per minute) in the 70S ribosomal fraction after ribonuclease treatment and hot trichloroacetic acid precipitation to exclude unreacted phenylalanyl-tRNA.

**Tetracycline inhibits protein synthesis**. Therefore it will prevent the reaction mixture from synthesizing $^{14}$C-labelled polyphenylalanine (Fig. 8.8, tetracycline-treated mix). This will lead to a significantly lower amount of radioactivity detected alongside the 70S ribosomal assembly within a sucrose density gradient column. Table 8.1 shows the effect of various tetracycline drugs on the rate of $^{14}$C-polyphenylalanine synthesis for reaction mixtures [3]. Every single drug inhibits $^{14}$C-polyphenylalanine synthesis, and therefore it is more informative to report the concentration of tetracycline required for half-maximal inhibition of $^{14}$C-polyphenylalanine synthesis ($ID_{50}$).

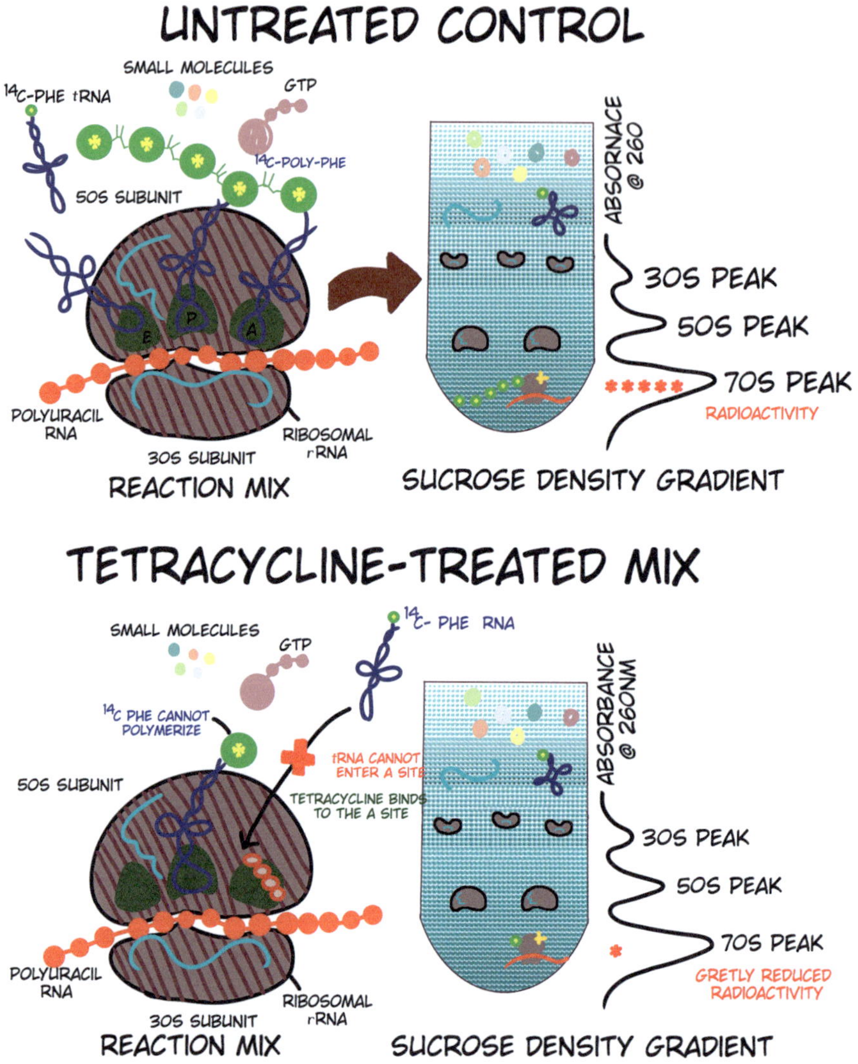


**Fig. 8.8** Illustration of the reaction mixture used to confirm **tetracycline inhibits protein synthesis**. Recall that protein synthesis begins with fMet-tRNA binding to the P-site. Therefore a low level of radioactivity even in the tetracycline-treated reaction mix is expected. Note that this experiment only confirms that tetracycline inhibits protein synthesis. It **DOES NOT** indicate that tetracycline inhibits protein synthesis by binding to the A-site, even though this binding is depicted in the diagram. Another experiment is required to confirm this mechanism and is described in Sect. 8.3.5

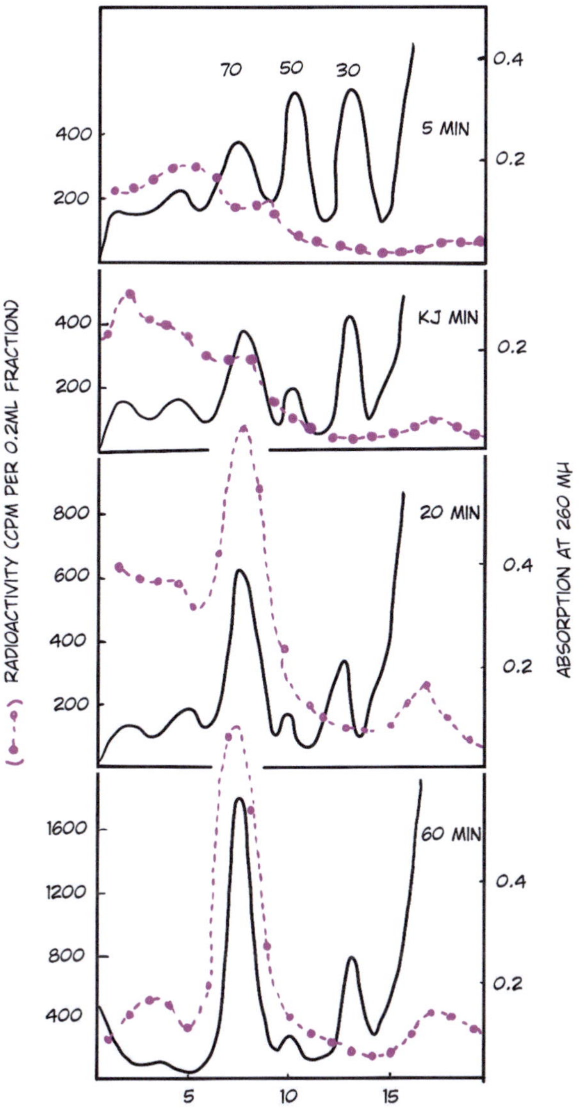


**Fig. 8.9 Poly-$^{14}$C-phenylalanine synthesis from a Polyuracil (-(UUU)$_n$-) template in an ex vivo reaction mix**, monitored over time. Initially (**t=5 min**), the bacterial ribosome is disassembled and displays separate 30S, 50S, and 70S peaks on a sucrose density gradient (ribosomal concentration estimated from rRNA absorbance at 260 nm). The 70S peak (representing an assembled ribosome) is the minor constituent and possesses radioactivity not significantly different from the baseline, indicating protein synthesis has not yet started. As the reaction proceeds (**t=20min, 30 min**), the 70S peak increases in magnitude, indicating assembly of the bacterial ribosome from 30S and 50S constituents. Counts per minute (cpm) also increase over time in the fraction containing the 70S ribosome, indicating protein synthesis is occurring. From this data, the rate of ex vivo protein synthesis per ribosome was calculated to be 280 residues hour$^{-1}$ ribosome$^{-1}$

**Technique 8.1**

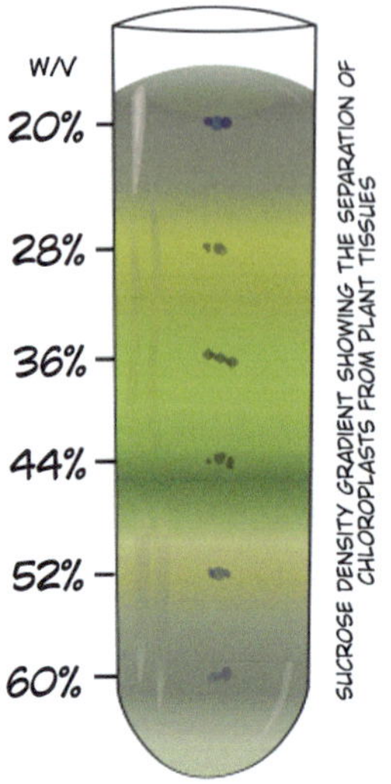


**Sucrose density gradient centrifugation** is a useful technique for partitioning biological macromolecules like DNA, RNA, proteins, and even organelles. The technique begins with the creation of a density gradient: layers of sucrose solutions ranging from ≥60% sucrose at the bottom of the centrifuge tube to ≤ 20% at the top are carefully prepared. The viscosity of sucrose solutions prevents them from simply diffusing into one another. Greater concentrations of sucrose also have higher densities. A low→high density gradient is therefore created from the top→bottom of the tube. Samples are placed at the top or bottom of the tube, depending on experiment, before centrifugation is performed. The constituents of the sample are then separated based on their size, shape, and density. Typically, larger molecules (like 70S ribosomes) sediment toward the bottom, and smaller molecules (like 16S ribosomes, individual proteins, small molecules, etc.) sediment progressively toward the top.

► **Remark**

Although a radioassay using $^{14}C$-labelled polyphenylalanine is described here, a variety of other techniques can be used to track ribosomal polyphenylalanine synthesis. Unlabelled polyphenylalanine can be quantified using **2D PAGE**, **thin-layer chromatography**, or simply **mass spectrometry** (preferably LC-MS).

### 8.3.5 Binding to the A-Site

Tetracycline binds to the A-site of the ribosome, preventing aminoacylated tRNA from binding with the mRNA / 70S ribosomal complex. This conclusion was reached from the following series of observations and inferences:

1. Tetracycline completely inhibits protein synthesis in a ribosomal reaction mix. This was described in detail in Sect. 8.3.4.
2. However, tetracycline only inhibits the 70S ribosomal binding with phenylalanyl-tRNA by **50%** (Fig. 8.10, inset **1** and **2**).

**Inference 8.1** There must exist **two separate binding sites for phenylalanyl-tRNA**, only one of which is the target of tetracycline. Today we know these sites as the **A- and P-sites.**

3. Tetracycline does not inhibit the binding of polyphenylalanyl-tRNA to the ribosome (Fig. 8.10, inset **3**). Note that polyphenylalanyl-tRNA can be chemically synthesized before the start of the experiment.

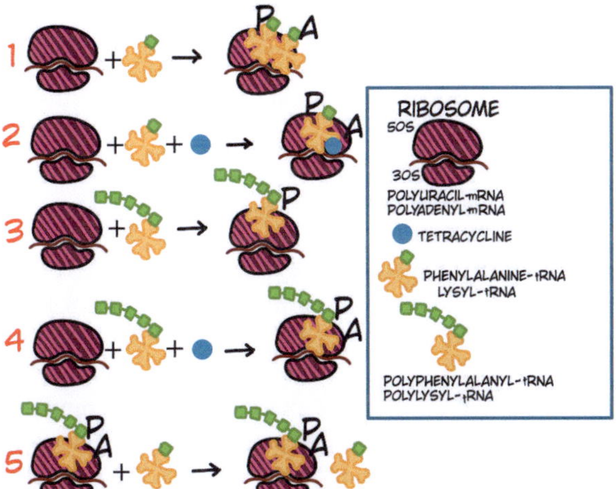


**Fig. 8.10** Observations that lead to the conclusion that **tetracycline binds to the A-site** on the 70S ribosome. (**1**): Untreated ribosomes showing 100% binding to (phe)-tRNA. (**2**): Tetracycline-treated ribosomes showing 50% binding to (phe)tRNA. (**3**): Untreated ribosomes showing 100% binding to poly(phe)-tRNA. (**4**): Tetracycline-treated ribosomes showing 100% binding to poly(phe)-tRNA. (**5**): Tetracycline- and poly(phe)-tRNA-treated ribosomes showing no binding to (phe)-tRNA

4. Ribosomes treated with polyphenylalanyl-tRNA and tetracycline (Fig. 8.10, inset **4**) no longer bind to any phenylalanyl-tRNA (Fig. 8.10, inset **5**).

**Inference 8.2 From observation 4:** Poly(phe)-tRNA must share one of the sites (phe)-tRNA binds to (**the A- or P-sites**).

**Inference 8.3 From observation 3:** This site is the one not affected by tetracycline (**the P-site**).

**Inference 8.4** From inferences 7.2 and 7.3, **tetracycline must inhibit tRNA-ribosome binding at the A-site**.

All the observations described were obtained through an intricate series of experiments performed by several independent workers [8, 9, 10]. Understanding all of their work is beyond the scope of this book, but the reader is encouraged to explore the references provided. If so inclined, the reader may even try to independently design experiments that could verify the claims discussed here.

### 8.3.6 Binding to the 30S Subunit

Tetracycline binds to several subunits (**S4, S5, S7, S15/16, S17**) (individual protein/rRNA chains) within the **30S ribosomal subunit** (Fig. 8.11). This was confirmed using **photoincorporation** studies [11] (Fig. 8.12). $^{3}$H-tetracycline was incubated with 70S ribosomes and exposed to a short, concentrated burst of UV rays. Tetracycline is a chromophore. The energy it absorbs from UV rays will cause chemical alterations within the tetracycline molecule. In particular, it can cause tetracycline to covalently link to protein/rRNA residues immediately surrounding it. Individual protein chains that constitute the ribosome can then be separated using a sucrose density gradient or a 2D SDS PAGE. The covalently linked $^{3}$H-tetracycline will remain bonded to its respective chains through all separation procedures, even if the 70S ribosome is disassembled. Therefore, the presence of radioactivity on individual rRNA/protein chains indicates that they form the tetracycline binding site.

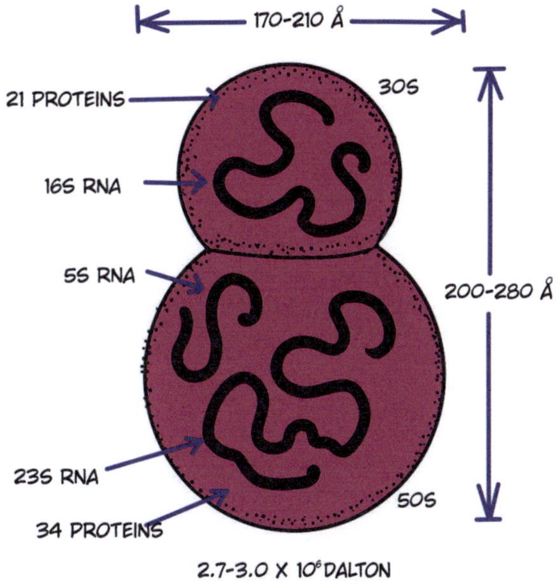


**Fig. 8.11** The 70S bacterial ribosome

It should be noted that when exposed to UV light, tetracycline can also form **photodegradation products**, some of which will contain the radioactive $^3$H atom. These products can migrate a considerable distance before covalently bonding to protein or rRNA residues. Care must be taken to minimize the creation of such molecules.

### 8.3.7 Challenging the Consensus

▶ **Remark**
Based on experimental observations, the existence of the A-, P-, and E-sites was inferred long before the crystal structure of the ribosome was solved in 2006 [12]. Even today, we are still not entirely sure which ribosomal substructures perform which functions. This only complicates the process of understanding anti-ribosomal antibiotics' mechanisms of action.

All the experiments described so far within this section have shaped the current consensus on the mechanism of action of tetracycline against bacterial pathogens. While it is undisputed that tetracycline inhibits protein synthesis, the consensus on the specific mechanisms through which it interacts with the ribosome have recently been challenged [13] for the following reasons:

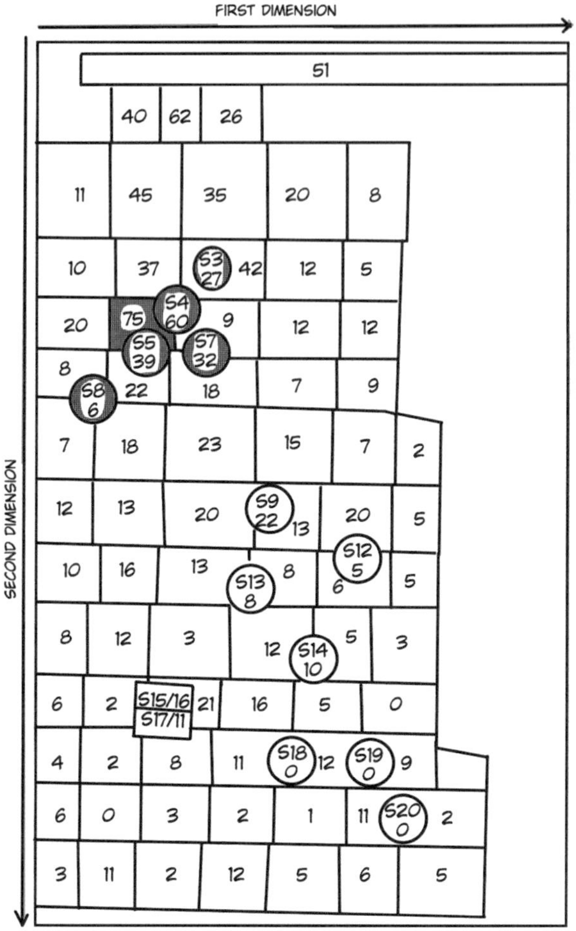


**Fig. 8.12 2D urea-PAGE of $^{3}$H-labelled and photoincorporated tetracycline [11]**. The gel was segmented after running, and the radioactivity of each section was assayed (*numbers in italic* represent counts per minute). Higher counts represent greater regions of radioactivity, and therefore greater tetracycline photoincorporation and consequently regions of tetracycline binding. Goldman et al. performed the experiment on intact 70S ribosomes but did not report a 2D PAGE for the 50S subunit, presumably because binding was only observed on the 30S subunit. Goldman et al. have also not provided the original 2D urea-PAGE image in their publication and have instead only supplied this diagram

1. Various studies reporting photoincorporation, X-ray crystallographic, Fenton chemistry, and chemical footprinting experiments have produced different and occasionally conflicting reports. Crystallization cannot distinguish between specific and nonspecific tetracycline binding sites. The 30S ribosome was crystallized with multiple tetracycline molecules binding to it for this reason [14] (Fig. 8.13).
2. Previous studies had reported tetracycline binding interactions with **both the 16S and 23S rRNAs** [15].
3. A study reporting in vivo experiments suggested that tetracycline inhibits rRNA synthesis [16]. Unfortunately, the community appears to have largely ignored this evidence.
4. Tetracycline is effective against a variety of **non-bacterial infections**, such as those caused by viruses and protozoa that lack mitochondria.

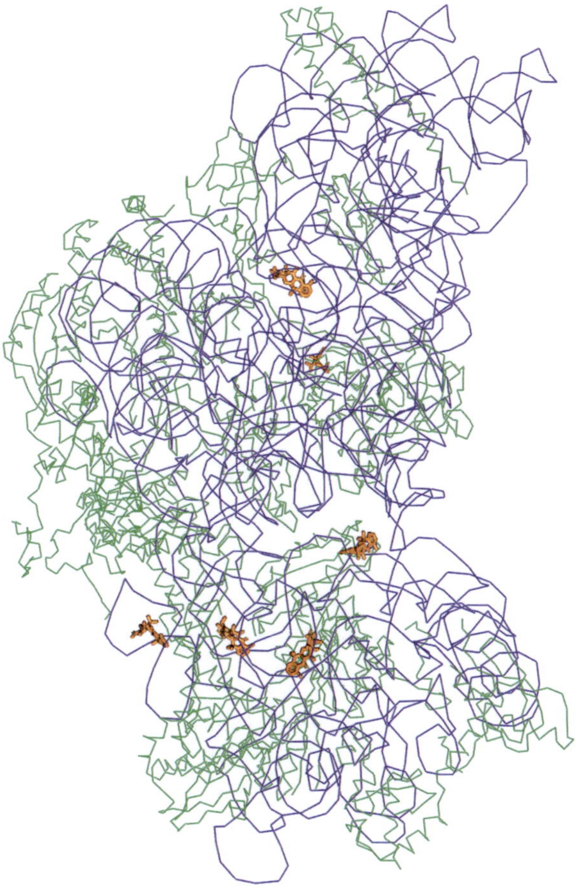

**Fig. 8.13 Crystal structure of the ribosomal 30S subunit co-crystallized with tetracycline.** PDB ID: 1i97 [14]. Protein subunits are colored green. The rRNA backbone is colored purple. Six tetracycline molecules (orange) can be seen bound to this ribosome. From this data alone, it is impossible to say which tetracycline molecule is specifically bound, and which tetracycline molecules are nonspecifically bound

5. Tetracycline is also effective at treating **noninfectious conditions**. Long-term tetracycline therapy is effective at controlling Crohn's disease.

These observations indicate that tetracycline may have **multiple mechanisms of action** against multiple kinds of diseases.

## 8.4 Tetracycline Resistance Mechanisms

Bacteria acquire tetracycline resistance through at least five mechanisms [17]:

1. **Innate mechanisms**: Some bacteria are naturally more resistant to tetracycline due to differences in the permeability of their cell membranes.

2. **Ribosome protection proteins**: These proteins bind to the ribosome, removing tetracycline from its binding site. At least 12 classes of such proteins have been reported.
3. **FAD-requiring monooxygenases**: These enzymes hydroxylate the tetracycline molecule and promote its degradation via non-enzymatic decomposition. These monooxygenases require oxygen to function, limiting their usefulness to aerobic pathogens only.
4. **16S rRNA mutants**: Such mutations confer resistance by altering the rRNA-tetracycline binding site.
5. **Efflux pumps**: At least 28 different classes of efflux pumps have been documented for tetracycline. Read Sect. 3.4.3 for more details.

### Technique 8.2

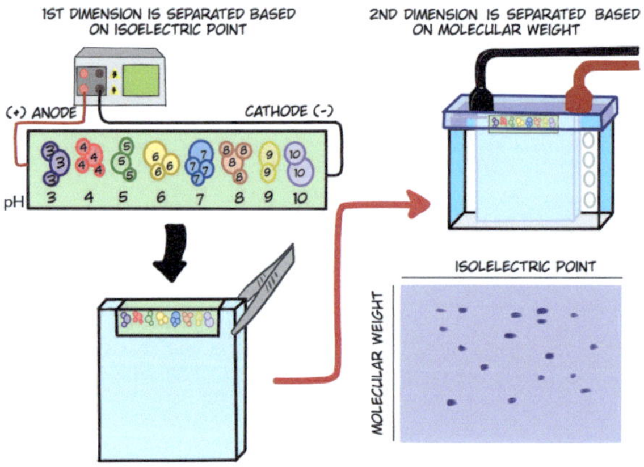


**2-dimensional polyacrylamide gel electrophoresis (2D-PAGE)** is a technique used to separate macromolecules, but usually proteins, based on two physical attributes. Proteins are usually separated based on their **isoelectric point (pI)** and their **size (molecular weight)**.

Proteins are first separated based on their isoelectric points using cylindrical polyacrylamide gels with an **immobilized pH gradient**. The buffering molecule (immobiline) is covalently linked to the acrylamide substrate while casting the gel. Their immobility prevents them from migrating under an electric field, maintaining the pH gradient.

Proteins are loaded at any point along this cylinder and allowed to migrate along the electric field. Negatively charged proteins will migrate toward the cathode. Positively charged proteins will migrate toward the anode. Proteins will display a net neutral charge when they reach their unique isoelectric point, and will occupy a unique position in the column, after which they will migrate no further.

Multiple proteins can possess very similar isoelectric points and will still need to be resolved further. The second dimension involves a **denaturing urea PAGE** to separate proteins based on their molecular weights, performed on the proteins separated by their pIs. The cylindrical polyacrylamide gel is simply loaded onto a urea/polyacrylamide gel and placed in an electric field.

Several hundred individual proteins can be resolved on a single 2D PAGE gel, making it a powerful tool for understanding complex protein assemblies such as the ribosome.

## 8.5 Problems

### Problem 8.1

An experimental tetracycline derivative (magicycline) specifically binds to the ribosome with a 1:1 stoichiometry. It does not display any nonspecific binding. Design a simple experiment to demonstrate that this is true.

### Problem 8.2

You have prepared a reaction mix containing ribosomes capable of cell-free protein synthesis. Use this system to confirm the mechanisms of action of experimental antibiotics suspected to:

1. Prevent the 70S ribosome from assembling around mRNA.
2. Block the exit of tRNA from the ribosome.
3. Block the polypeptide exit tunnel.

### Problem 8.3

Your guide hands you an experimental antibiotic that inhibits ribosomal protein synthesis. Your guide believes it functions by binding exclusively to the ribosomal P-site, whereas an experienced postdoc claims it binds to both the A-site and P-site. Describe a series of observations and inferences you would need to make to confirm which hypothesis is correct. You need not describe full experiments.

### Problem 8.4

An FAD-requiring monooxygenase is suspected to hydrolyze tetracycline. Design a simple experiment to confirm that this is the case.

## References


1. Pautke C, Vogt S, Kreutzer K, Haczek C, Wexel G, Kolk A, Imhoff AB, Zitzelsberger H, Milz S, Tischer T (2010) Characterization of eight different tetracyclines: advances in fluorescence bone labeling. J Anatomy 217(1):76–82
2. Armelagos GJ, Kolbacher K, Collins K, Cook J, Krafeld-Daugherty M (2001) Tetracycline consumption in prehistory. In Tetracyclines in biology, chemistry and medicine, pp 219–236. Springer
3. Tritton TR (1977) Ribosome-tetracycline interactions. Biochemistry 16(18):4133–4138
4. Maxwell IH (1968) Studies of the binding of tetracycline to ribosomes in vitro. Mol Pharmacol 4(1):25–37
5. Staehelin T, Maglott DR (1971) [47] preparation of Escherichia coli ribosomal subunits active in polypeptide synthesis. In: Methods in enzymology, vol 20, pp 449–456. Elsevier
6. Zubay G (1962) The isolation and fractionation of soluble ribonucleic acid. J Mol Biol 4(5):347–356
7. Vögeli G, Grosjean H, Söll D (1975) A method for the isolation of specific tRNA precursors. Proc Natl Acad Sci 72(12):4790–4794
8. Suarez G, Nathans D (1965) Inhibition of aminacyl-sRNA binding to ribosomes by tetracycline. Biochem Biophys Res Commn 18(5-6):743–750
9. Gottesman ME (1967) Reaction of ribosome-bound peptidyl transfer ribonucleic acid with aminoacyl transfer ribonucleic acid or puromycin. J Biol Chem 242(23):5564–5571
10. Sarkar S, Thach RE (1968) Inhibition of formylmethionyl-transfer RNA binding to ribosomes by tetracycline. Proc Natl Acad Sci 60(4):1479–1486. https://www.pnas.org/doi/abs/10.1073/pnas.60.4.1479
11. Goldman RA, Hasan T, Hall CC, Strycharz WA, Cooperman BS (1983) Photoincorporation of tetracycline into Escherichia coli ribosomes. Identification of the major proteins photolabeled by native tetracycline and tetracycline photoproducts and implications for the inhibitory action of tetracycline on protein synthesis. Biochemistry 22(2):359–368
12. Selmer M, Dunham CM, Murphy IV FV, Weixlbaumer A, Petry S, Kelley AC, Weir JR, Ramakrishnan V (2006) Structure of the 70 s ribosome complexed with mRNA and tRNA. Science 313(5795):1935–1942
13. Chukwudi CU (2016) rRNA binding sites and the molecular mechanism of action of the tetracyclines. Antimicrobial Agents Chemotherapy 60(8):4433–4441
14. Pioletti M, Schlünzen F, Harms J, Zarivach R, Glühmann M, Avila H, Bashan A, Bartels H, Auerbach T, Jacobi C, et al. (2001) Crystal structures of complexes of the small ribosomal subunit with tetracycline, edeine and IF3. EMBO J 20(8):1829–1839
15. Day LE (1966) Tetracycline inhibition of cell-free protein synthesis ii. effect of the binding of tetracycline to the components of the system. J Bacteriol 92(1):197–203
16. Atherly AG (1974) Specific inhibition of ribosomal RNA synthesis in Escherichia coli by tetracycline. Cell 3(2):145–151
17. Nguyen F, Starosta AL, Arenz S, Sohmen D, Dönhöfer A, Wilson DN (2014) Tetracycline antibiotics and resistance mechanisms. Biol Chem 395(5):559–575

# Streptomycin

# 9

Deepesh Nagarajan

**Abstract**

Streptomycin is an aminoglycoside antibiotic isolated from *Streptomyces griseus*. Streptomycin was initially used to treat tuberculosis before more effective drugs entered the clinic. Streptomycin's mechanism of action involves binding to the 30S subunit of the bacterial ribosome and causing misreadings in the genetic code. Cell-free ribosomal reaction mixtures capable of *in vitro* translation, using a mixture of radiolabeled and non-radiolabeled aminoacyl t-RNA, can be used to record the frequency of codon misreadings. Streptomycin resistance mechanisms involve mutations to the S12 ribosomal subunit, streptomycin-inactivating enzymes, and multidrug efflux pumps.

**Keywords**

Streptomycin · Aminoglycoside · Codon misreading · Antibiotic resistance

Streptomycin is an **aminoglycoside antibiotic** used to treat a number of bacterial infections, including tuberculosis, neonatal sepsis, peritonitis, endocarditis, brucellosis, plague, and rat bite fever.

D. Nagarajan (✉)
Department of Biotechnology, M.S. Ramaiah University of Applied Sciences, Bangalore, India

Department of Microbiology, St. Xavier's College, Mumbai, India
e-mail: deepeshn.bt.ls@msruas.ac.in; deepesh.nagarajan@xaviers.edu

© The Editor(s) (if applicable) and The Author(s), under exclusive license to Springer Nature Singapore Pte Ltd. 2024

D. Nagarajan (ed.), *Antibiotics and Their Mechanisms of Action*,
https://doi.org/10.1007/978-981-97-6851-6_9

## 9.1 History

Streptomycin was isolated in 1943 from *Streptomyces griseus*, an actinomycete. Credit for its discovery is jointly shared by **Selman Waksman** and **Albert Schatz**, the former's PhD student. Streptomycin was the second major antibiotic discovered after penicillin and filled important clinical niches penicillin left uncovered.

> It is almost impossible to exaggerate the importance of this discovery. Streptomycin not only filled a large number of Gram negative gaps in the spectrum of penicillin, including efficacy in plague, but proved effective in the treatment of tuberculosis. Patients even began to recover from tubercular meningitis, until then the most inevitably and regularly fatal of all bacterial infections.
> ~**L.P. Garrod** [1]
> (British bacteriologist)

Between 1946 and 1948, the Medical Research Council (MRC) Tuberculosis Research Unit (UK) conducted a randomized curative trial for streptomycin as a treatment against pulmonary tuberculosis [2]. This trial is considered to be the first of its kind; however it was neither double-blind nor placebo-controlled. Unfortunately, *Mycobacterium tuberculosis* rapidly evolves resistance against streptomycin. Streptomycin is therefore used in combination with other drugs (such as isoniazid, p-aminosalicylic acid, and ethambutol) as part of multidrug treatment against tuberculosis.

▶ **Remark**

A **single blind clinical trial** involves blinding a given patient to the knowledge of whether the drug they are consuming is real or a placebo. Doctors will not be blinded.

A **double blind clinical trial** involves blinding both the doctor(s) and a given patient to the knowledge of whether the drug the given patient is consuming is real or a placebo. A third party not directly involved in treating the patients will retain this knowledge.

## 9.2 Aminoglycoside Antibiotics

The term "aminoglycoside" is used to refer to any antibiotic containing one or more **amino sugar** moieties (Fig. 9.1). Streptomycin was the first antibiotic discovered in this class. Others soon followed (Table 9.1).

Although initially popular, since the 1980s the medical community has shifted away from the clinical use of aminoglycosides due to both their toxicity (nephrotoxicity and ototoxicity, rarely neuromuscular blockade, and hypersensitivity reactions [4]), and the availability of third-generation cephalosporins, carbapenems, and fluoroquinolones [3]. Increasing resistance to aminoglycoside replacements, however, has led to renewed interest in these drugs. Arbekacin and plazomicin are novel

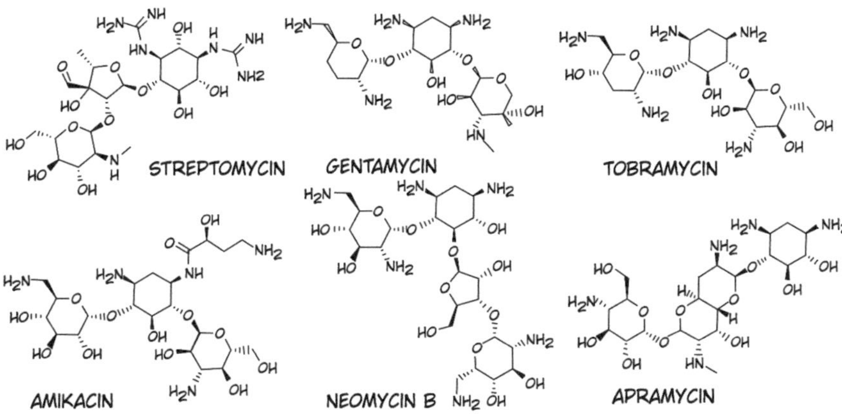


**Fig. 9.1 Structures of representative aminoglycoside antibiotics**. Note the amine ($NH_2$) groups in place of hydroxyls in the amino sugars

**Table 9.1 Aminoglycoside antibiotics**: their names, origin, and date of discovery/synthesis [3]

| Aminoglycoside | Origin | Year |
|---|---|---|
| Streptomycin | *Streptomyces griseus* | 1944 |
| Neomycin | *Streptomyces fradiae* | 1949 |
| Kanamycin | *Streptomyces kanamyceticus* | 1957 |
| Gentamicin | *Marantochloa purpurea* | 1963 |
| Netilmicin | Chemical derivative | 1967 |
| Tobramycin | *Streptoalloteichus tenebrarius* | 1967 |
| Amikacin | Chemical derivative | 1972 |
| Arbekacin | Chemical derivative | 1973 |
| Plazomicin | Chemical derivative | 2012 |

aminoglycosides designed with the intention of overcoming resistance mechanisms common to the aminoglycoside class.

## 9.3 Mechanism of Action

Streptomycin binds to the **30S subunit** of the ribosome and causes **misreadings in the genetic code**.

▶ **Remark**

Two isomers of streptomycin exist in nature, each with their own mechanism of action. While **streptomycin A** causes misreadings in the genetic code, **streptomycin B** acts by inhibiting peptidoglycan synthesis. Streptomycin A is the only clinically used form of streptomycin and is therefore simply referred to as "streptomycin."

Streptomycin–ribosome binding can be demonstrated very easily using a thermal shift assay as described for penicillin in Sect. 3.3.2 and tetracycline in Sect. 8.3.4. The specific ribosomal subunits streptomycin binds to can be traced using photoincorporation experiments [5] as described for tetracycline in Sect. 8.3.6. For brevity, similar experiments will not be repeated here.

▶ **Remark**

Unlike tetracycline, streptomycin is not naturally photosensitive. A $^3$**H-labeled photoactivated analog of streptomycin** (photo-Sm [5]) therefore has to be used for photoincorporation studies.

Streptomycin-induced codon misreading can be demonstrated using a cell-free ribosomal reaction mix designed to synthesize polyphenylalanine from polyuracil (-(UUU)$_n$-) mRNA (see Sect. 8.3.1 and Fig. 8.8).

This system can be modified to elucidate streptomycin's mechanism of action with little effort (Fig. 9.2) using the following protocol:

1. Prepare 20 separate aliquots of the standard cell-free ribosomal reaction mixture (containing unlabeled Phe-tRNA). Each aliquot corresponds to an amino acid.
2. Divide these aliquots into two subaliquots each (40 aliquots total). Of these two subaliquots, one serves as a control (no streptomycin), and the other is used for the experiment (streptomycin-added).
3. Add $^{14}$**C-labeled aminoacyl-tRNA**, containing the respective amino acid, to each of the 40 aliquots.
4. Incubate all aliquots to allow for the translation of polyuracil (-(UUU)$_n$-).
5. After incubation treat all 40 aliquots with trichloroacetic acid (TCA) to precipitate out macromolecules. Polypeptides will precipitate out, whereas aminoacylated-tRNA will not.
6. For a given streptomycin-treated aliquot, corresponding to a given radiolabeled amino acid, radioactivity in the TCA precipitate indicates incorporation of the radiolabeled amino acid into the polypeptide.

**Inference 9.1** If a radiolabeled amino acid that is NOT Phe is incorporated into the polypeptide, then it indicates streptomycin-induced codon misreading.

7. Likewise, for a given non-streptomycin-treated aliquot corresponding to the same amino acid, one should expect no radioactivity in the TCA precipitate.

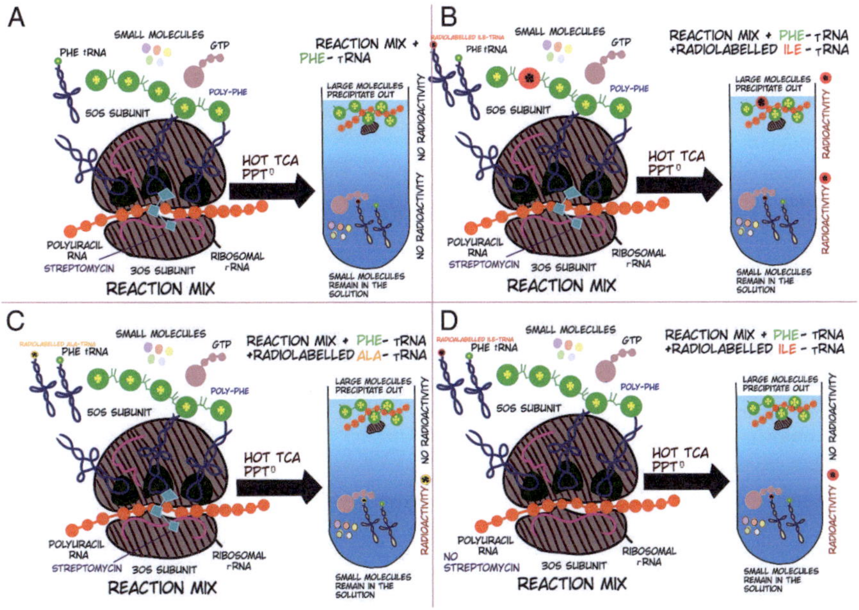


**Fig. 9.2 Cell-free ribosomal reaction mix adapted to determine streptomycin's mechanism of action**. **(a): Reaction mix + Phe-tRNA + streptomycin**: standard, unmodified reaction mix with no radiolabels. Phe is expected to be incorporated into the polypeptide (poly-Phe) whether streptomycin is present or absent. **(b): Reaction mix + Phe-tRNA + radiolabeled Ala-tRNA + streptomycin**: streptomycin causes specific codon misreadings. It does not cause the incorporation of Ala in place of Phe during the translation of polyuracil. No radioactivity will be observed in the trichloroacetic acid (TCA) precipitate. Radioactivity will be observed in the soluble fraction, simply because radiolabeled Ala-tRNA was added to the reaction mixture. **(c): Reaction mix + Phe-tRNA + radiolabeled Ile-tRNA+ streptomycin**: streptomycin specifically incorporates **Ile**, **Leu**, and **Ser** in the place of Phe through codon misreadings during the translation of polyuracil. Radioactivity will be observed in the trichloroacetic acid (TCA) precipitate. Radioactivity will also be observed in the soluble fraction. **(d): Reaction mix + Phe-tRNA + radiolabeled Ile-tRNA**: the same as **(c)** but lacking streptomycin. A simple control to confirm that codon misreading observed in **(c)** was caused by streptomycin alone

**Inference 9.2** For a given amino acid that is NOT Phe, observing radioactivity in the streptomycin-treated aliquot, while also observing no radioactivity in the non-streptomycin-treated aliquot, confirms that codon misreading was caused by streptomycin alone.

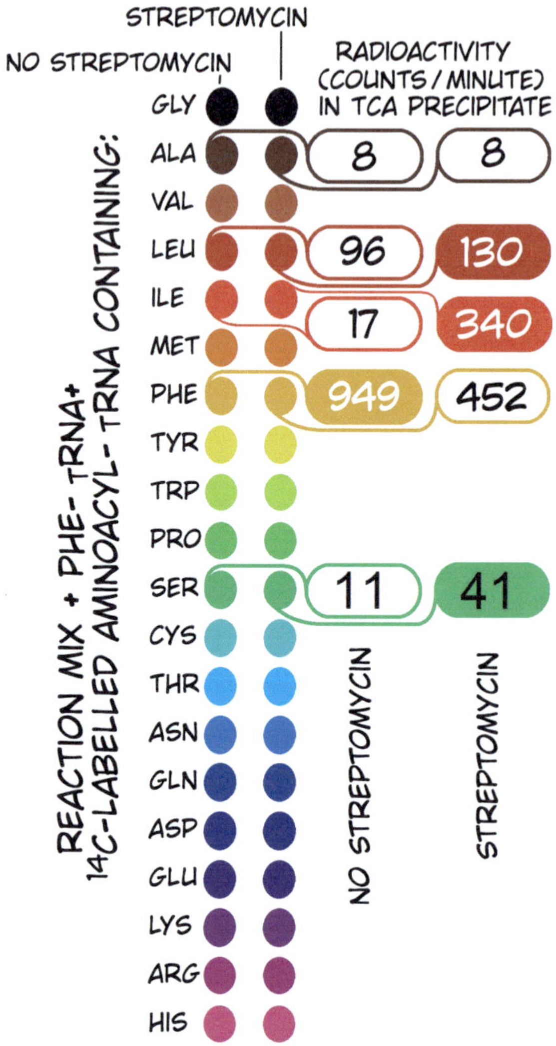


**Fig. 9.3 Select observations that confirm streptomycin's mechanism of action via codon misreading**. Protocol discussed in text. Streptomycin causes codon misreading and the incorporation of $^{14}$C-labeled **Leu**, **Ile**, and **Ser** into poly-Phe synthesized using a cell-free ribosomal reaction mix. In all three cases, radioactivity (measures in counts per minute/cpm) in the streptomycin-treated aliquots is higher than that in the non-streptomycin-treated aliquots, confirming streptomycin-induced codon misreading. Streptomycin does not cause the erroneous incorporation of **Ala** into poly-Phe; therefore both the streptomycin treated and non-streptomycin-treated aliquots have the same levels of radioactivity. Streptomycin causes a decrease in the rate of incorporation of Phe into poly-Phe, as evidenced by the lower radioactivity measured in the streptomycin-treated aliquot. Data for all amino acids can be found in the original publication [6]

Using the above protocol, streptomycin was found to cause specific codon misreadings of polyuracil (-(UUU)$_n$-) for three amino acids: **Ile**, **Leu**, and **Ser** [6] (Fig. 9.3).

▶ **Remark**

Protein function is entirely dependent on protein structure, while protein structure is entirely dependent on protein sequence. Even a single amino acid mutation on a protein sequence can cause the protein structure to misfold and lose its function.

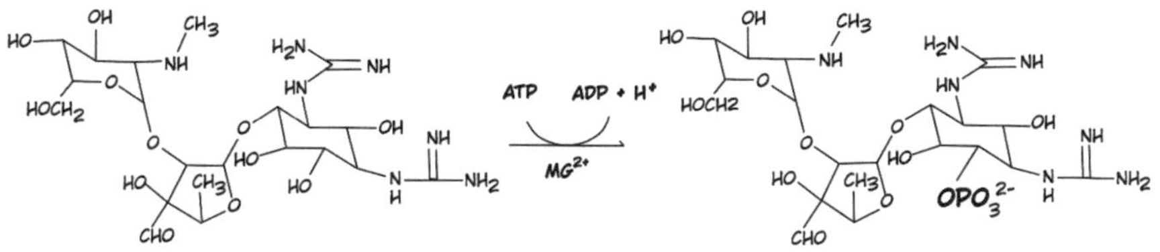


**Fig. 9.4** **Reaction catalyzed by aminoglycoside phosphotransferase**

## 9.4 Streptomycin Resistance Mechanisms

Resistance to streptomycin occurs due to the following mechanisms:

1. Mutations to the gene encoding the protein for the **S12 ribosomal subunit** (rpsL), found within the 30S subunit, and at the 50S/30S interface [7]
2. Mutations within the **16S rRNA** [8]
3. **Streptomycin-inactivating enzymes**: strA and strB [9]. Aminoglycoside phosphotransferase [10], which phosphorylates and inactivates streptomycin (Fig. 9.4)
4. **Efflux pumps**; read Sect. 3.4.3 for more details

## 9.5 Problems

**Problem 9.1**

How would you confirm the mechanism of action for streptomycin B?

**Problem 9.2**

You plan to elucidate the mechanisms of action of streptomycin derivatives using the adapted cell-free ribosomal reaction mix, as described in Sect. 9.3. You plan to test all 20 amino acids for misreadings against a polyuracil mRNA template. Unfortunately, your guide informs you that he will be unable to afford 20 separate radiolabeled aminoacyl-tRNAs for your experiments. The best he can do is buying you one such tRNA.
Which radiolabeled aminoacyl-tRNA do you choose?
Describe your amended experimental protocol.

**Problem 9.3**

Your guide hands you an experimental aminoglycoside (lambdamycin) that he suspects causes histidine misreadings in the genetic code. Unfortunately, your guide can no longer supply you with radiolabeled compounds. Your guide suggests that you design an experiment using modern molecular biology techniques, rather than using a cell-free ribosomal reaction mix, to confirm the mechanism of action.

Describe the design of such an experiment.

**Problem 9.4**

You have isolated a potential aminoglycoside phosphotransferase from a streptomycin-resistant strain of *E. coli*. Describe an experiment to confirm its enzymatic activity.

## References


1. Wainwright M (1991) Streptomycin: discovery and resultant controversy. History Phil Life Sci, 97–124
2. Metcalfe NH (2011) Sir Geoffrey Marshall (1887–1982): respiratory physician, catalyst for anesthesia development, doctor to both prime minster and king, and World War I barge commander. J Med Biography 19(1):10–14
3. Krause KM, Serio AW, Kane TR, Connolly LE (2016) Aminoglycosides: an overview. Cold Spring Harbor Perspect Med 6(6):a027029
4. Gonzalez LS III, Spencer J (1998) Aminoglycosides: a practical review. Am Family Physician 58(8):1811
5. Girshovich AS, Bochkareva ES, Ovchinnikov YA (1976) Identification of components of the streptomycin-binding center of E. coli MRE 600 ribosomes by photo-affinity labelling. Mol General Genet MGG 144(2):205–212
6. Davies J, Gilbert W, Gorini L (1964) Streptomycin, suppression, and the code. Proc Natl Acad Sci 51(5):883–890
7. Springer B, Kidan YG, Prammananan T, Ellrott K, Bottger EC, Sander P (2001) Mechanisms of streptomycin resistance: selection of mutations in the 16S rRNA gene conferring resistance. Antimicrobial Agents Chemotherapy 45(10):2877–2884
8. Cooksey RC, Morlock GP, McQueen A, Glickman SE, Crawford JT (1996) Characterization of streptomycin resistance mechanisms among mycobacterium tuberculosis isolates from patients in New York city. Antimicrobial Agents Chemotherapy 40(5):1186–1188
9. Sundin GW, Bender CL (1996) Dissemination of the strA-strB streptomycin-resistance genes among commensal and pathogenic bacteria from humans, animals, and plants. Mol Ecol 5(1):133–143
10. Ashenafi M, Ammosova T, Nekhai S, Byrnes WM (2017) Purification and characterization of aminoglycoside phosphotransferase APH (6)-Id, a streptomycin-inactivating enzyme. Mol Cellular Biochem 387(1):207–216

# Chloramphenicol

# 10

Deepesh Nagarajan

**Abstract**

Chloramphenicol is an antiribosomal antibiotic that was isolated from *Streptomyces venezuelae*. It was initially used as a broad spectrum antibiotic before being withdrawn from clinical use in the West, due to concerns that it may increase the risk of aplastic anemia. Chloramphenicol remains in use in other parts of the world. Chloramphenicol is a structural analog of aminoacyl-tRNA, which initially hinted at its mechanism of action. Its mechanism of action involves inhibition of protein synthesis by binding to the bacterial ribosome and inhibiting the formation of the peptide bond. Chloramphenicol accomplishes this by inhibiting ribosomal peptidyl transferase activity. This can be demonstrated using a peptidyl transferase reaction mix containing ribosomal subunits and $^{35}$S-CAACCA-formyl-methionine. Puromycin, another protein synthesis inhibitor, can be used to confirm the chloramphenicol-induced inhibition of peptide bond formation. Chloramphenicol resistance is caused by mutations to the 23S rRNA, chloramphenicol acetyltransferases, 3-O-phosphorylation of the chloramphenicol molecule, and by multidrug efflux pumps.

**Keywords**

Chloramphenicol · PPuromycin · Aplastic anemia · Drug resistance

D. Nagarajan (✉)
Department of Biotechnology, M.S. Ramaiah University of Applied Sciences, Bangalore, India

Department of Microbiology, St. Xavier's College, Mumbai, India
e-mail: deepeshn.bt.ls@msruas.ac.in; deepesh.nagarajan@xaviers.edu

© The Editor(s) (if applicable) and The Author(s), under exclusive license to Springer Nature Singapore Pte Ltd. 2024

D. Nagarajan (ed.), *Antibiotics and Their Mechanisms of Action*,
https://doi.org/10.1007/978-981-97-6851-6_10

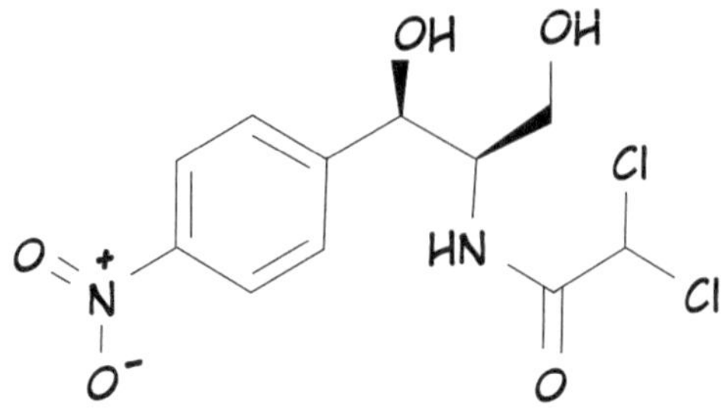


**Fig. 10.1 Structure of chloramphenicol**. Initially the structure was accepted with much reservation as a nitro group has previously not been observed on a natural chemical compound [1]

Chloramphenicol is a broad spectrum, bacteriostatic antibiotic used to treat a wide range of gram-positive and gram-negative infections. Topically applied chloramphenicol is particularly useful for the treatment of ophthalmic infections such as conjunctivitis (infection and inflammation of the transparent membrane lining the eyeball), endophthalmitis (infection of the aqueous and vitreous fluids), and blepharitis (inflammation of the eyelids) as well as otitis externa (infection of the external ear). Chloramphenicol initially enjoyed widespread use but has been phased out of use in some countries due to concerns about its toxicity and potential carcinogenicity, some of which are not well founded.

## 10.1 History

Chloramphenicol was discovered in 1947 by researchers working at **Parke-Davis**. It was isolated from *Streptomyces venezuelae*, an actinomycete species. In 1949, **Mildred Rebstock et al.** from Parke-Davis reported chloramphenicol's chemical structure [1] (Fig. 10.1). It was initially used to treat typhoid, but the rise of chloramphenicol-resistant *S. typhi* in the 1980s relegated it to other roles.

## 10.2 Toxicity, Disuse, and Resurgence

Chloramphenicol use may lead to **aplastic anemia** (a deficiency of all types of blood cells, Fig. 10.2), bone marrow suppression, and leukemia as side effects. Chloramphenicol use may also lead to **gray baby syndrome** in newborn infants. Prominent symptoms include a gray coloration of the skin and cyanosis (blue discoloration of the lips and skin). These side effects have led to chloramphenicol being phased out in North America in favor of new generation fluoroquinolones [2].

Data collected in California in the 1960s indicated that the risk of aplastic anemia occurring after consuming 7.5 g of chloramphenicol was 1:21,671, or 11.5x higher compared the chloramphenicol-exclusive baseline of 1:250,000 [3]. This data was later contradicted by chloramphenicol usage trends in Hong Kong from the 1980s, where usage per capita is 11-442x greater than in western countries, but whose death rate from aplastic anemia is considerably lower [4]. The risk of blood dyscrasia

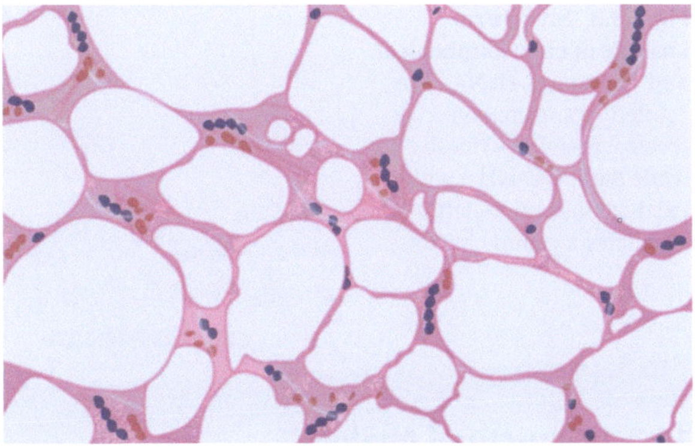

**Fig. 10.2** **Bone marrow section of a patient with aplastic anemia**, showing a lack of cellular matter and increased spaces corresponding to fat deposits (Artist's Impression)

(all blood-related diseases) after topical chloramphenicol use is only 1:20 million, which is far lower than the risk of penicillin-induced anaphylaxis of 1:100,000 [2]. A reconsideration for the use of chloramphenicol in North America is therefore warranted.

▶ **Remark**
The **ESKAPE pathogen family** consists of *Enterococcus faecium*, *Staphylococcus aureus*, *Klebsiella pneumoniae*, *Acinetobacter baumannii*, *Pseudomonas aeruginosa*, and *Enterobacter spps*. Strains belonging to these species comprise the vast majority of drug-resistant and nosocomial infections, especially in ICUs.

Chloramphenicol's alleged toxic effects may soon be ignored in favor of its efficacy against multidrug-resistant pathogens. MIC data shows that chloramphenicol is largely effective against ESKAPE pathogens and meticillin-resistant *S. aureus* (MRSA) [5].

## 10.3 Mechanism of Action

**Chloramphenicol inhibits protein synthesis** by binding to the bacterial ribosome and **inhibiting the formation of the peptide bond** (ribosomal peptidyl transferase) (Fig. 8.2).

Chloramphenicol-ribosome binding can very easily be demonstrated using a thermal shift assay as described for penicillin in Sect. 3.3.2 and tetracycline in Sect. 8.3.4. Likewise, chloramphenicol's inhibition of protein synthesis can very easily be demonstrated using the cell-free ribosomal reaction mix described for tetracycline in Sect. 8.3.1 (Fig. 8.8) or using radiolabelled tracers to track DNA/RNA/protein synthesis as described in Sect. 6.4 (Fig. 6.3). For brevity, similar experiments will not be repeated here.

Demonstrating that chloramphenicol inhibits ribosomal peptidyl transferase, however, requires new experiments.

**Fig. 10.3 Structural analogy of chloramphenicol and aminoacyl-tRNA**. The "curled" conformation (center) resembles ribose, while the (O=C-NH-) within the dichloracetyl moiety resembles a peptide bond

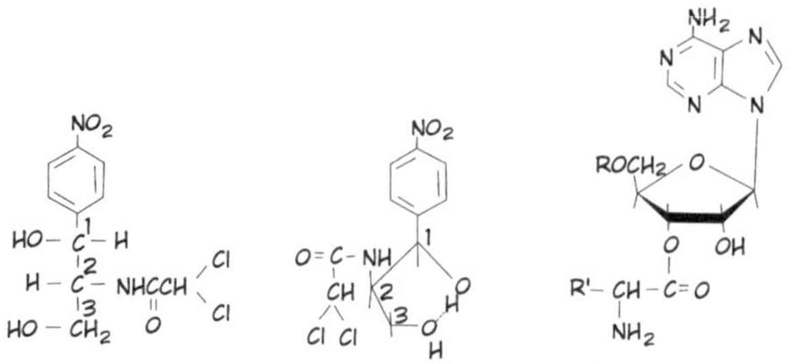


## 10.3.1 Structural Analogy

Chloramphenicol was first noticed to be a **structural analog of aminoacyl-tRNA** in 1966, while its mechanism of action was still being elucidated [6] (Fig. 10.3). The linear molecule is capable of adopting a **pseudo-cyclic "curled" conformation** in solution. This conformation is stabilized by a hydrogen bond between two hydroxyl groups, making the molecule resemble the site of attachment of the amino acid/peptide on tRNA. Recall how penicillin is a structural analogue of the terminal (D-ala)-(D-ala) on the pentapeptide linkage and was therefore suspected to be a transpeptidase inhibitor (see Sect. 6.4). Similarly, chloramphenicol's structural analogy to aminoacyl-tRNA, and the fact that it contained a structure analogous to the peptide bond (O=C-NH-) within its dichloroacetyl moiety, raised suspicions that it inhibited peptide bond synthesis via competitive inhibition.

## 10.3.2 Inhibition of Peptide Bond Formation

In order to study the inhibition of peptide bond formation, a model system that isolates the ribosomal peptidyl transferase center from all the other functional centers is needed. Such a system can be created with the following components:

1. 70S ribosomes or even just **50S ribosomal subunits**. The 30S subunit is unnecessary.
2. **CAACCA-formyl-methionine**, derived from fmet-tRNA.
3. **Puromycin** (see Infobox 10.4).
4. $\mathbf{Mg^{2+}}$ and $\mathbf{K^{+}}$.
5. **Ethanol**, without which the peptidyl transferase reaction cannot occur within this system. It is possible that ethanol only facilitates the binding of CAACCA-fmet to the ribosomes, which does not happen under aqueous conditions.

Many constituents that would have otherwise been required for cell-free ribosomal protein synthesis (such as ATP and GTP) are not required here. Within this peptidyl transferase reaction mix, a peptide bond is formed between the C-terminal of CAACCA-formyl-methionine and the N-terminal analogue of

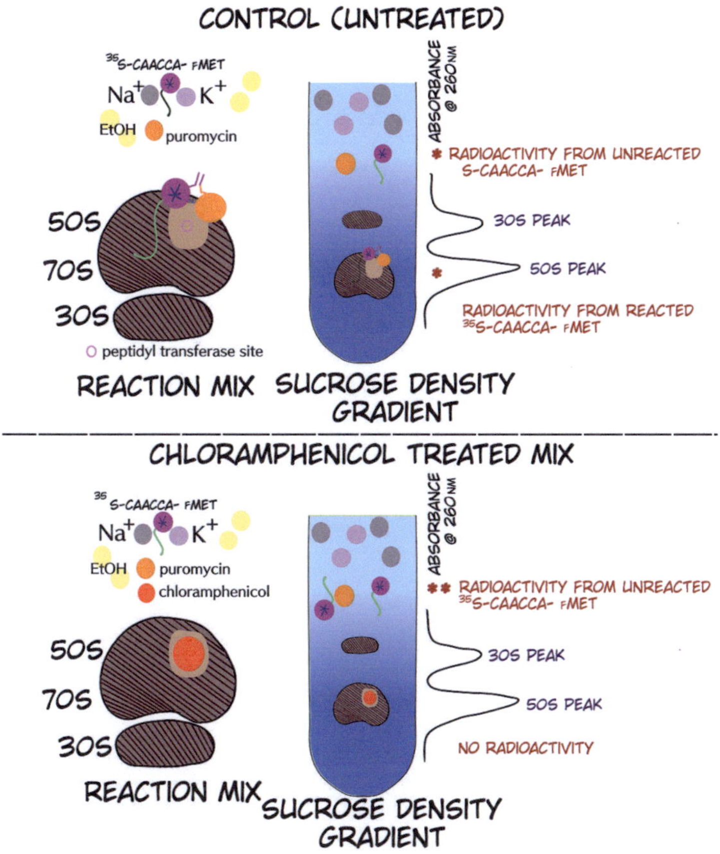


**Fig. 10.4** Illustration of the reaction mixture used to confirm that **chloramphenicol inhibits ribosomal peptidyl transferase activity**, using a modified cell-free ribosomal reaction mix as described in Sect. 10.3.2. Note that the 30S ribosomal subunit is not necessary for peptidyl transferase activity and is therefore shaded gray

puromycin. CAACCA-fmet-puromycin, analogous to peptidyl-puromycyl-tRNA, then remains attached to the 50S subunit of the ribosome. The methionine within CAACCA-fmet can be radiolabelled using $^{35}$S and tracked using **sucrose density gradient centrifugation**.

Chloramphenicol was observed to interfere with peptide bond formation within this peptidyl transferase reaction mix, as measured by a decrease in radioactivity (counts per minute) in the fraction containing 50S ribosomal subunits [7, 8] (Figs. 10.4, 10.5).

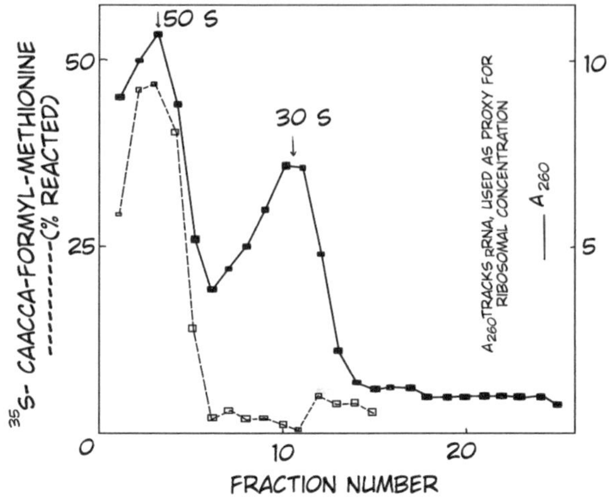


| CONDITION | $^{35}$S-CAACCA- FMET (% REACTED) |
|---|---|
| 70S RIBOSOMES | 77% |
| 50 SUBUNITS ONLY | 54% |
| 30S SUBUNNITS ONLY | -5% |
| 50S + 30S SUBUNITS | 52% |
| 70 RIBOSOMES + CHLORAMPPHENICOL (1MM) | 4% |

**Fig. 10.5** **Chloramphenicol inhibits ribosomal peptidyl transferase activity**. **(Graph)** Sucrose density gradient centrifugation of a peptidyl transferase reaction mix containing 70S ribosomes, $^{35}$S-CAACCA-formyl-methionine, and puromycin. Radioactivity is observed on the 50S subunit, indicating the formation of a peptide bond between $^{35}$S-CAACCA-fmet and puromycin. **(Table)** Percent $^{35}$S-CAACCA-fmet incorporation into the ribosome can be back-calculated from radioactivity (counts per minute) under different conditions. From these observations, we can infer that: (1) Only the 50S ribosome is required for peptidyl transferase activity [7]. (2) Chloramphenicol inhibits peptidyl transferase activity on the 70S ribosome [8] and therefore inhibits peptidyl transferase on the 50S ribosomal subunit by extension

**Caveats**: It should be noted that peptidyl transferase reaction mixtures depart significantly from natural or cell-free ribosomal protein synthesis in many respects:

1. Ethanol is required for peptide bond formation. Natural ribosomal systems function in aqueous media. The exact reason for this ethanol requirement has not yet been established.
2. The CAACCA-fmet-puromycin product is only loosely analogous to the natural tRNA-fmet-aminoacyl product.
3. CAACCA-fmet-puromycin does not depart the ribosome after synthesis, unlike peptidyl- puromycyl-tRNA (see Infobox 10.4).

These departures from the natural system may mean that chloramphenicol's elucidated mechanism of action may be significantly different from its in vivo mechanism of action.

## 10.4 Chloramphenicol Resistance Mechanisms

Chloramphenicol resistance occurs due to the following [10]:

1. **Chloramphenicol acetyltransferases (CATs)** that inactivate the drug molecule. CAT transfers the acetyl group from acetyl-CoA to chloramphenicol. This prevents chloramphenicol from binding to the ribosome (Fig. 10.6).
2. **3-O-phosphorylation** of the chloramphenicol molecule leading to its inactivation.
3. Reduced expression of **outer membrane proteins (OMPs)**, reducing the ability of chloramphenicol to reach the cytoplasm.
4. Mutations to, or methylation of, the chloramphenicol binding site on **23S rRNA** (with the 50S subunit).
5. **Efflux pumps**; read Sect. 3.4.3 for more details.

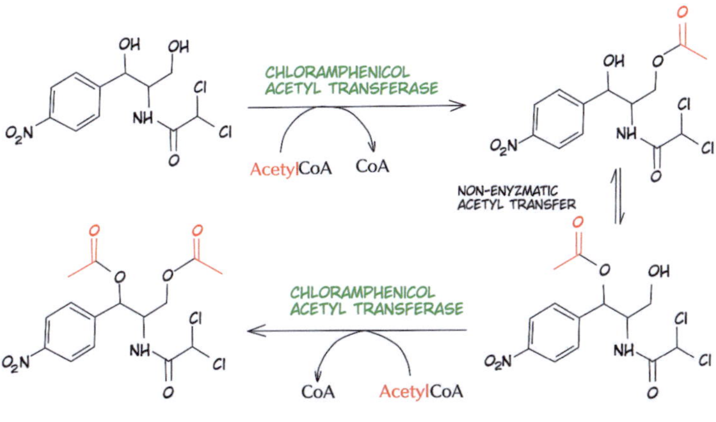


**Fig. 10.6 Reaction mechanism for chloramphenicol acetyltransferases** [9]. The acetyl molecules (red) change the chemical structure of chloramphenicol and prevent it from binding to the bacterial ribosome

**Infobox 10.1**

**Understanding the mechanism of action of chloramphenicol using puromycin**

Understanding the mechanism of action of chloramphenicol using puromycin

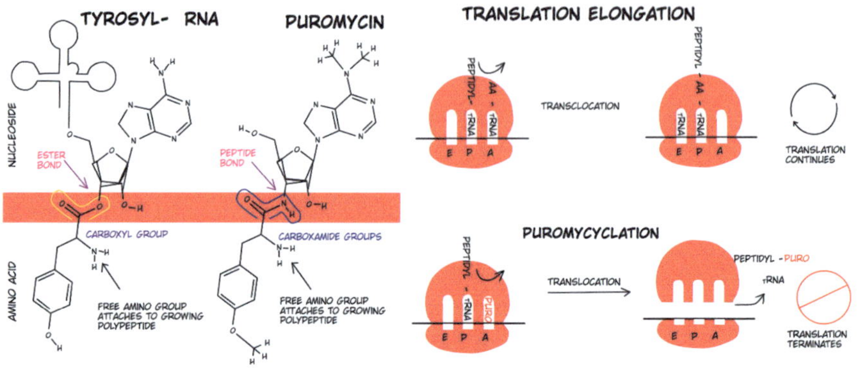


Puromycin is a naturally found antibiotic and a protein synthesis inhibitor [11]. Like chloramphenicol, it is an aminoacyl-tRNA analogue. Its mechanism of action involves entering the ribosome at the A-site and incorporating its amino acid analogue (methyltyrosine) into the C-terminus of the growing polypeptide chain. Methyltyrosine lacks an analogue to the C-terminus: It possesses a carboxamide ($CONH_2$) rather than a carboxylate ($COO^-$) at this position. Therefore other amino acids cannot be incorporated into the growing polypeptide chain after puromycin. Translation ends after puromycin incorporation into the growing polypeptide chain, leading to peptidyl-puromycyl-tRNA release from the ribosome.

## 10.5 Problems

**Problem 10.1**

Should chloramphenicol have been withdrawn from use in North America? Why or why not?

**Problem 10.2**

You are preparing to test the in vitro efficacy of chloramphenicol derivatives using a modified cell-free ribosomal reaction mix, as described in Sect. 10.3.2. Unfortunately, your clumsy project assistant spills your modified reaction mix, losing it all in the process. Your project assistant apologizes and suggests using a standard cell-free ribosomal reaction mix you used to study tetracycline derivatives (Sect. 8.3.4) for your current experiments on the chloramphenicol

derivatives. She believes both reaction mixtures are interchangeable for this particular purpose.
Is your project assistant correct? Why or why not?

**Problem 10.3**

Propose experiments to confirm puromycin's mechanism of action.

**Problem 10.4**

You are preparing to test the in vitro mechanism of action of chloramphenicol derivatives using a modified cell-free ribosomal reaction mix, as described in Sect. 10.3.2. Unfortunately, you do not have $^{35}$S-CAACCA-fmet in stock. You only have regular, unlabelled CAACCA-fmet. However, you have the following radiolabelled compounds in stock:

1. $^{14}$C-puromycin
2. $^{3}$H-chloramphenicol
3. $^{32}$P-GTTGGT

Design an alternative experiment using one or more of the above labelled compounds to elucidate the mechanism of action of your chloramphenicol derivatives.

**Problem 10.5**

Design an experiment to confirm chloramphenicol acetyltransferase activity for a protein freshly isolated and purified from a chloramphenicol-resistant strain. You have access to a mass spectrometer (LC-MS).

## References

1. Rebstock MC, Crooks HM, Controulis J, Bartz QR (1949) Chloramphenicol (chloromycetin). 1 iv. 1a chemical studies. J Am Chem Soc 71(7):2458–2462
2. Isenberg SJ (2003) The fall and rise of chloramphenicol. J Am Assoc Pediatric Ophthalmol Strabismus {JAAPOS} 7(5):307–308
3. Wallerstein RO, Condit PK, Kasper CK, Brown JW, Morrison FR (1969) Statewide study of chloramphenicol therapy and fatal aplastic anemia. JAMA 208(11):2045–2050
4. Kumana CR, Li KY, Chau PY (1988) Worldwide variation in chloramphenicol utilization: should it cause concern? J Clin Pharmacol 28(12):1071–1075
5. Čivljak R, Giannella M, Di Bella S, Petrosillo N (2017) Could chloramphenicol be used against ESKAPE pathogens? a review of in vitro data in the literature from the 21st century. Expert Rev Anti-infective Therapy 12(2):249–264
6. Coutsogeorgopoulos C (1966) On the mechanism of action of chloramphenicol in protein synthesis. Biochimica et Biophysica Acta (BBA)-Nucleic Acids Protein Synthesis 129(1):214–217
7. Monro RE (1967) Catalysis of peptide bond formation by 50 s ribosomal subunits from Escherichia coli. J Mol Biol 26(1):147–151

8. Monro RE, Marcker KA (1967) Ribosome-catalysed reaction of puromycin with a formylmethionine-containing oligonucleotide. J Mol Biol 25(2):347–350
9. Elder FCT, Feil EJ, Pascoe B, Sheppard SK, Snape J, Gaze WH, Kasprzyk-Hordern B (2021) Stereoselective bacterial metabolism of antibiotics in environmental bacteria–a novel biochemical workflow. Front Microbiol, 738
10. Roberts MC, Schwarz S (2017) Tetracycline and chloramphenicol resistance mechanisms. In: Antimicrobial drug resistance, pp 231–243. Springer
11. Aviner R (2020) The science of puromycin: From studies of ribosome function to applications in biotechnology. Comput Struct Biotechnol J 18:1074–1083

# Antimetabolites

# 11

Deepesh Nagarajan

**Abstract**

Antimetabolites target the synthesis of a metabolite that is required for normal metabolism and survival of the pathogen. Sulfa drugs, such as sulfamethoxazole and sulfadiazine, in combination with trimethoprim are the most widely used antimetabolites. Sulfa drugs inhibit the folate biosynthesis pathway by targeting the enzyme dihydropteroate synthetase (DHPS). Trimethoprim targets the same pathway, but at a different enzyme called dihydrofolate reductase (DHFR). As such, both drugs display synergy that can easily be visualized using the strip diffusion test. The inhibition of DHFR and DHPS can be observed using a simple NADPH/$NADP^+$ colorimetric assay. Resistance to antimetabolites is conferred by mutations to DHPS and DHFR, DHFR overexpression, chromosomal recombination to incorporate new DHPS genes, and by multidrug efflux pumps.

**Keywords**

Antimetabolites · Sulfa drugs · Sulfamethoxazole · Trimethoprim · DHFR · DHPS · Drug resistance

Antimetabolites are antibiotics that target the synthesis of a metabolite that is essential for normal metabolism and survival of the pathogen. Antimetabolites act like **substrate analogues**: They structurally resemble a natural metabolite along a

D. Nagarajan (✉)
Department of Biotechnology, M.S. Ramaiah University of Applied Sciences, Bangalore, India

Department of Microbiology, St. Xavier's College, Mumbai, India
e-mail: deepeshn.bt.ls@msruas.ac.in; deepesh.nagarajan@xaviers.edu

© The Editor(s) (if applicable) and The Author(s), under exclusive license to Springer Nature Singapore Pte Ltd. 2024
D. Nagarajan (ed.), *Antibiotics and Their Mechanisms of Action*,
https://doi.org/10.1007/978-981-97-6851-6_11

critical anabolic pathway. **Competitive inhibition** occurs: Antimetabolites are able to bind to, and inhibit, enzymes along this pathway due to this structural similarity.

▶ **Remark**
The term "antimetabolite" should not be taken literally. By definition, **most antibiotics are antimetabolites**. Penicillin inhibits the synthesis of the bacterial cell wall, which itself is a metabolite. Rifampicin inhibits the synthesis of mRNA, which is also a metabolite. By convention, antimetabolites only **inhibit the synthesis of small molecules** that are precursors for the synthesis of larger, essential metabolites.

If antimetabolites specifically inhibit bacterial enzymes, they are useful as antibiotics. However, if antimetabolites inhibit human enzymes, they are still useful as **anticancer drugs**. Cancer cells rapidly divide, and therefore they always possess higher rates of metabolism compared to normal cells. Inhibiting all metabolism in the human body will therefore disproportionately affect cancer cells. It should be noted that other rapidly dividing cells in the human body like those in hair follicles, nail roots, and the bone marrow will also be affected by antimetabolites.

Unlike all other classes of antibiotics in clinical use today, antimetabolites are of entirely **synthetic origin**. They were not isolated from natural sources unlike penicillin (Sect. 3.1) or magainin (Sect. 5.1).

## 11.1 History

The history of antimetabolite drugs begins with experiments to determine the antibacterial activity of azo dyes (containing an **-N=N-** chromophore) [3]. In 1913, Philipp Eisenberg reported the antibacterial effects of the dye chrysoidine. Likewise Iwan Ostromislensky reported antibacterial effects of the dyes serenium and pyridium.

Building on this work, **Joseph Klarer** and **Fritz Mietzsch** [1] synthesized a range of such dyes that they handed over to **Gerhard Domagk** for further chemical modification and antimicrobial testing. In 1935, Domagk developed one such compound, KL695 (KL = Klarer), into KL730, which was renamed **prontosil** (Figs. 11.1, 11.2, 11.3). Prontosil was effective against gram-positive cocci but not against gram-negative enterobacteria.

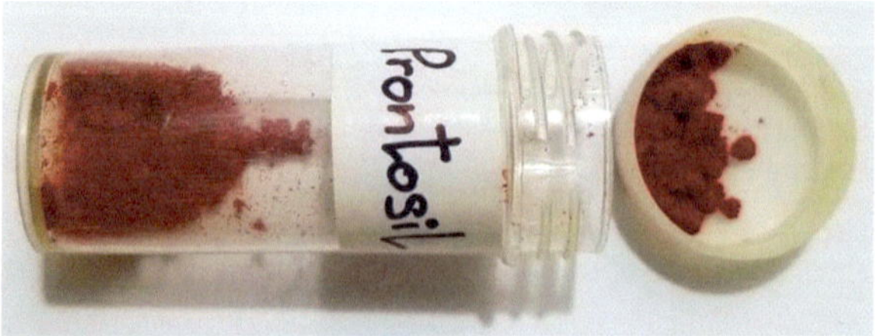


**Fig. 11.1** **Prontosil's dark red coloration** indicates that the antibiotic traces its lineage back to azo dyes

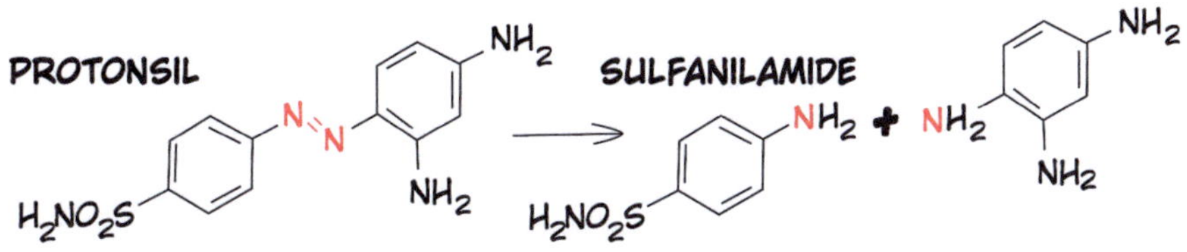


**Fig. 11.2** **Prontosil as a prodrug**. Prontosil is metabolized into sulfanilamide through a reduction of the azo bond. Sulfanilamide is therefore colorless

**Fig. 11.3** Prontosil along with its precursor (KL695) and its derivative (prontosil soluble). The azo **-N=N-** chromophore is responsible for the dark red coloration of these compounds

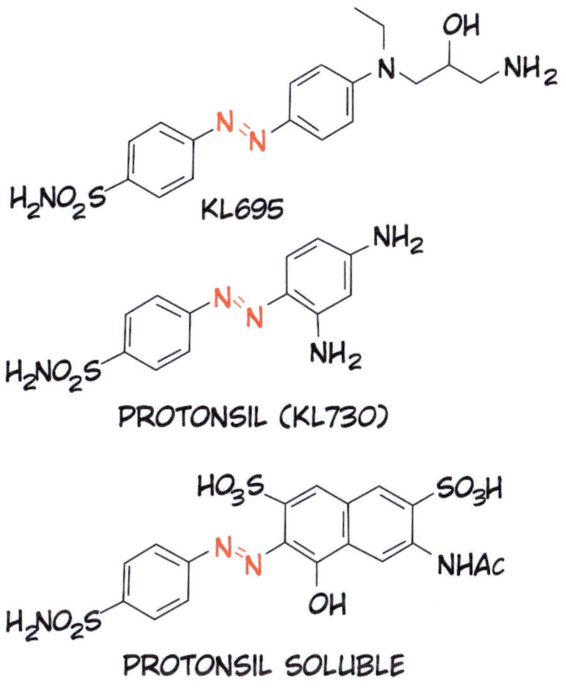


Prontosil (also named prontosil rubrum after its dark red coloration, Fig. 11.1) was relatively insoluble in water. This incentivized the development of **prontosil soluble**, which allowed for the rapid administration of the antibiotic in cases of serious disease.

Later work by **Ernest Fourneau** and **Jacques Tréfouël** in 1935 [2] showed that a prontosil metabolite, rather than prontosil itself, was the agent responsible for antimicrobial activity. This metabolite was named **sulfanilamide** and is formed through the reduction of the azo bond (**-N=N-**) within prontosil. It should be noted that as a prodrug, prontosil did not display in vitro activity but nevertheless displayed in vivo activity.

By the 1940s, sulfa drugs were well-established antibiotics. They were used by both sides during the Second World War to treat infected wounds (Fig. 11.4).

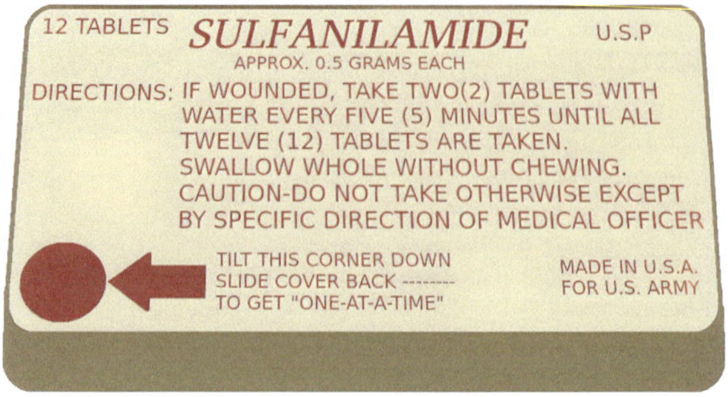


**Fig. 11.4** WW2-era sulfanilamide tablets issued to American frontline soldiers (artist's impression)

## 11.2 Sulfa Drugs

The advent of sulfanilamide leads to the **sulfa craze** of the 1930s, where manufacturers created and sold an immense number of sulfa formulations without any regulation. This inevitably leads to the **elixir sulfanilamide disaster** of 1937 [4], an incident where over 100 people were poisoned with diethylene glycol. More stringent regulations lead to most sulfa products being recalled for human use.

A list of sulfa antibiotics that are approved for clinical or veterinary use today is presented alongside. It should be noted that nonantibiotic (antidiabetic, anticancer, anticonvoluscant, antiretroviral, etc.) sulfa drugs are not listed here.

*Short acting sulfa drugs*:

1. **Sulfacetamide**: 10% topical lotion to treat acne and seborrheic dermatitis.
2. **Sulfadiazine**: Used alongside pyrimethamine to treat toxoplasmosis.
3. **Sulfadimidine**: Used to treat uncomplicated UTIs, prostatitis, and respiratory tract infections.
4. **Sulfafurazole**: Used to treat uncomplicated UTIs and systemic infections. Erythromycin/sulfafurazole is sold as pediazole, used to treat acute otitis media in children.
5. **Sulfisomidine**: Closely related to sulfadimidine.

*Intermediate acting sulfa drugs*:

1. **Sulfamethoxazole**: Extensively used to treat UTIs, bronchitis, and prostatitis.
2. **Sulfamoxole**: Used for treating pediatric infections.
3. **Sulfanitran**: Used as a feed additive for chickens to control infections caused by **Coccidioides spps**.

*Long acting sulfa drugs*:

1. **Sulfadimethoxine**: Used for treating intestinal coccidioisis in cats and dogs.

2. **Sulfamethoxypyridazine**: Used for treating vaginal irritation, severe acute thrush, and dermatitis herpetiformis as an alternative to dapsone.
3. **Sulfametoxydiazine**: Used as a leprostatic agent and in the treatment of UTIs.

*Ultra-long acting sulfa drugs*:

1. **Sulfadoxine**: Used in combination with pyrimethamine to treat malaria.
2. **Sulfametopyrazine**: Used to treat chronic bronchitis, UTIs, and malaria.
3. **Terephtyl**: Used on susceptible strains.

Although all the sulfa drugs listed above are approved for clinical or veterinary use, in practice most have been set aside in favor of more effective antibiotics developed much later. Sulfametopyrazine, for example, is only marketed in Thailand and Ireland today. Of all the drugs listed, **sulfamethoxazole** remains the most relevant.

Sulfa drugs are sometimes used in combination with **trimethoprim**, another antibiotic that targets an enzyme along the same metabolic pathway.

## 11.3 Mechanism of Action

Understanding the importance of folate for the metabolism of essential molecules is a prerequisite to understanding the mechanism of action of sulfa drugs.

### 11.3.1 Folate Metabolism

Folate (or vitamin B9) is an essential micronutrient required for both human health and bacterial growth. A folate deficiency in humans leads to megaloblastic anemia, heart palpitations, dyspnea, and many other conditions.

Figure 11.5 places **folate metabolism** in a broader context, showing its relationship with other essential metabolic pathways [5]. These pathways are mostly conserved across all kingdoms of life. However, unlike humans, bacteria are also capable of synthesizing dihydrofolate using the **folate biosynthesis pathway**.

The folate pathway is required to methylate uridine monophosphate (UMP), converting it into thymidine monophosphate (TMP) via the **thymidylate cycle**, without which DNA synthesis cannot occur.

Likewise, the folate pathway is required for the synthesis of adenosine monophosphate (AMP) and guanosine monophosphate (GMP) via the **purine biosynthetic cycle**, without which DNA and RNA synthesis cannot occur.

Finally, the folate pathway is required for the **methionine cycle** responsible for synthesizing methionine and cysteine. Methionine, of course, is the start codon required for the synthesis of all proteins.

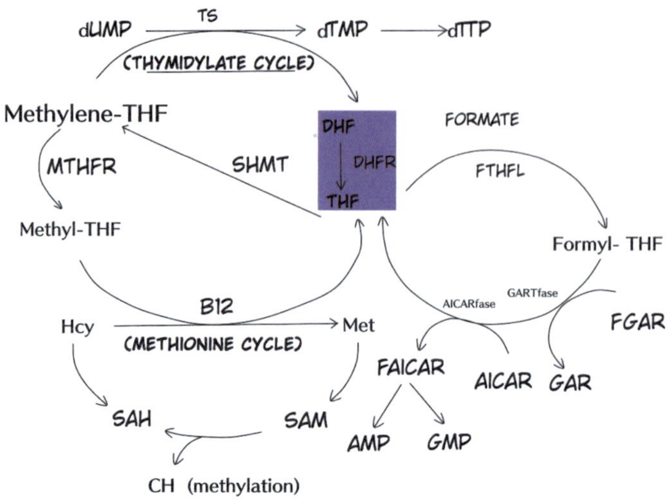


**Fig. 11.5** **Folate metabolism** placed in context with other essential metabolic pathways [5]. Only a portion of the **folate biosynthesis pathway** is shown here (highlighted in violet). **DHF**: dihydrofolate, **THF**: tetrahydrofolate, **DHFR**: dihydrofolate reductase

### 11.3.2 Folate Biosynthesis Pathway

Unlike humans, bacteria are capable of synthesizing folate using the folate biosynthesis pathway. Several enzymes along this pathway are required to convert **guanosine triphosphate (GTP)** into **dihydrofolate** and then **tetrahydrofolate** (Fig. 11.6), both of which are required as substrates for other essential metabolic pathways (Fig. 11.5).

Of particular note are two enzymes along this pathway: **dihydropteroate synthetase (DHPS)** and **dihydrofolate reductase (DHFR)**.

▶ **Remark**
In the scientific literature, the terms *dihydropteroate synthetase* and *dihydropteroate synthase* are used interchangeably.

**DHPS** catalyzes the formation of dihydropteroate from hydroxymethyl-7,8 dihydropterin pyrophosphate and **para-amino benzoic acid**. Sulfa drugs act like **substrate analogs**. Sulfamethozaxile and sulfanilamide, for example, **structurally resemble PABA** (Infobox 11.1): They all share a common benzamine ring (Fig. 11.6, in red). This high degree of structural similarity allows sulfa drugs to competitively inhibit DHPS by mimicking the substrate, attaching to the binding site, and preventing the **real** substrate from binding and undergoing catalysis.

**DHFR** catalyzes the reduction of dihydrofolic acid to tetrahydrofolic acid, utilizing **NADPH** in the process. Like sulfa drugs, trimethoprim acts through competitive inhibition. Trimethoprim competes against dihydrofolic acid for the

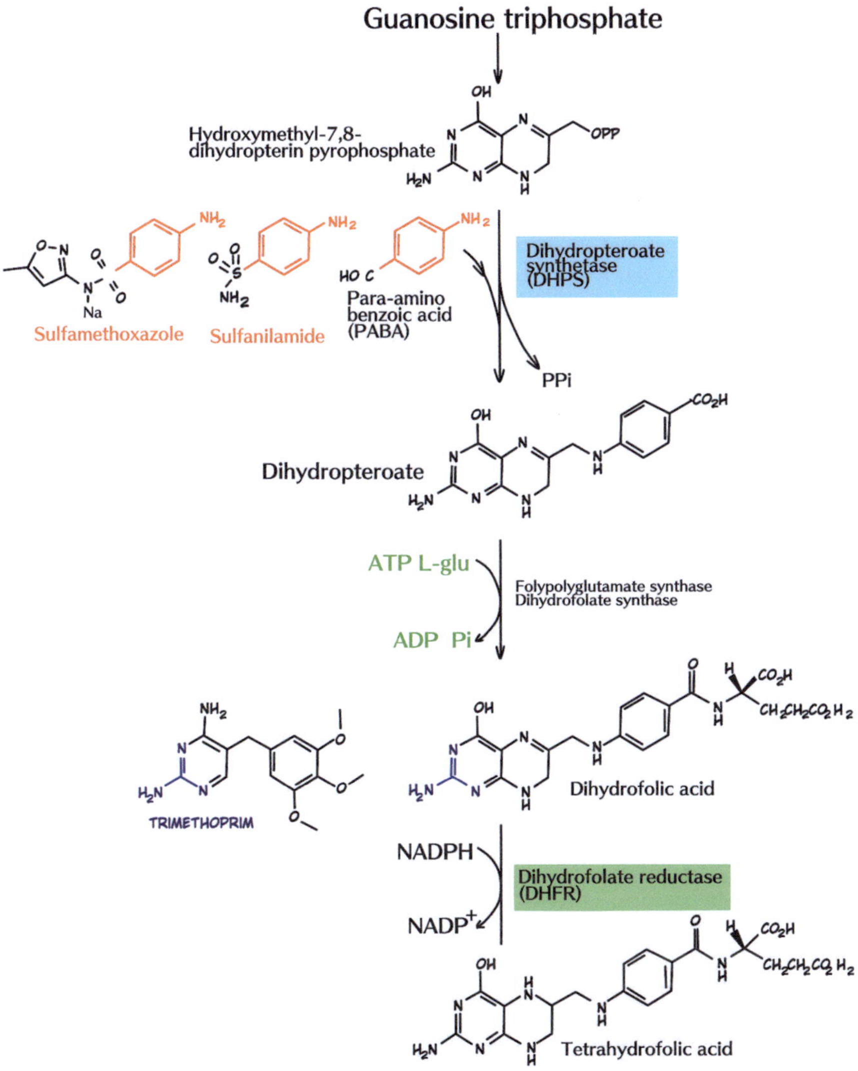


**Fig. 11.6 Folate biosynthesis pathway** dihydrofolate and tetrafolate are synthesized from guanosine triphosphate (GTP) in several steps

DHFR binding site, thereby inhibiting the enzyme's activity. Unlike sulfa drugs, trimethoprim shares markedly **less substrate analogy**, only sharing a common guanido group with dihydrofolic acid (Fig. 11.6, in blue).

Sulfamethoxazole and trimethoprim act on enzymes along the **same metabolic pathway**. Therefore, they both exhibit **synergy** when used in combination. Bactrim (1 part trimethoprim/5 parts sulfamethoxazole) is routinely used to treat urinary tract infections.

### 11.3.3 Inhibition of DHFR and DHPS

Trimethoprim's effect on the activity of dihydrofolate can easily be observed using a simple **colorimetric assay**. NADPH absorbs light at 340 nm, whereas $NADP^+$ does not. Likewise, NADPH fluoresces at 445 nm when excited at 340 nm, whereas $NADP^+$ does not.

To assay DHFR activity, a simple reaction mixture containing known quantities of dihydrofolic acid and NADPH can be created. Absorbance at 340 nm must be tracked the instant DHFR is introduced. A **decrease in absorbance at 340 nm over time** would indicate $NADP^+$ production, therefore NADPH utilization, therefore **DHFR activity** (Fig. 11.7).

**Trimethoprim inhibits DHFR activity**, and therefore the **absorbance at 340 nm is not expected to change** if trimethoprim was added to the aforementioned reaction mix before the addition of DHFR.

**Sulfa drugs' inhibition of DHPS** can also be easily tracked using the **same colorimetric reaction** setup [6]. An expanded reaction mix containing all the substrates and enzymes needed for 2 steps of the folate pathway starting at DHPS is required. DHPS lies 2 reactions above DHFR on the folate biosynthesis pathway. The product of DHPS will be needed for the creation of substrate for DHFR, which will then be reduced using NADPH. DHPS inhibitors will therefore also halt the oxidation of NADPH in this expanded reaction mix and can therefore be tracked using absorbance at 340 nm.

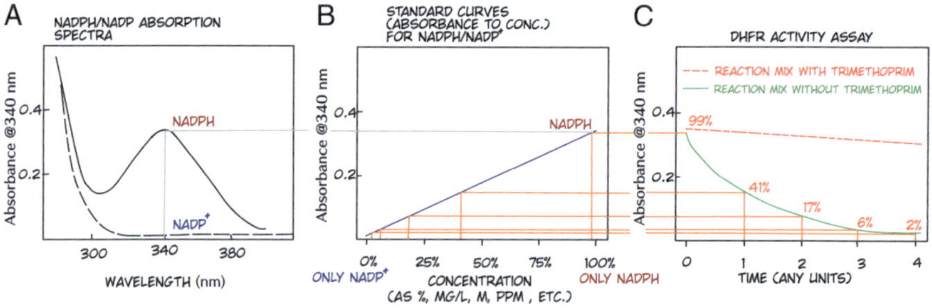


**Fig. 11.7** An example **colorimetric assay** used to visualize **the inhibition of DHFR by trimethoprim**, as described in the text. **(a)** NADPH shows an absorption maxima at 340 nm, whereas $NADP^+$ does not. **(b)** By the Beer–Lambert law, the absorbance of a compound is linearly proportional to its concentration. Therefore, a standard curve of concentration vs. absorbance can be plotted for an experimentally relevant range of NADPH concentrations. **(c)** This standard curve can then be used to calculate the concentrations of NADPH at different time intervals during a DHFR activity assay. Reaction mixtures (as described in the text) with and without trimethoprim added are expected to utilize NADPH differently and therefore display different absorbance vs. time curves

Technique 11.1

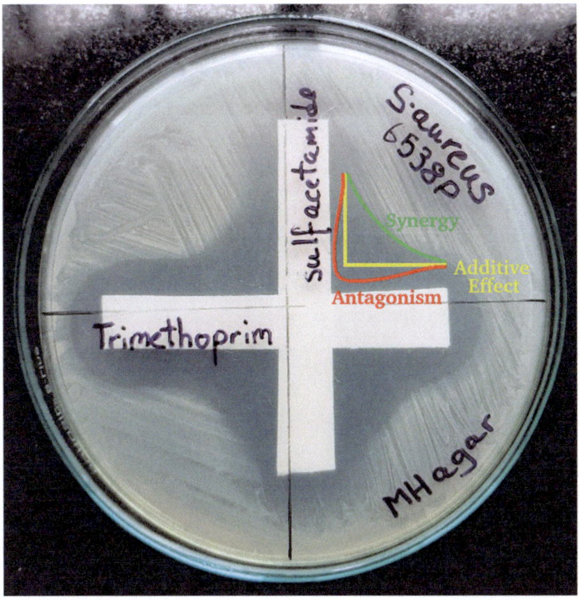


How can one determine whether two antibiotics exhibit synergy when used in combination? This can easily be answered using the **strip diffusion test**. Using sulfamethoxazole and trimethoprim as examples, two strips of paper impregnated with a solution of each antibiotic are prepared. These strips are laid out in an "X" pattern on a lawn of sensitive bacteria (usually *E. coli* grown on Mueller Hinton (MH) agar. After overnight incubation, the pattern of inhibition on the MH agar plate is observed:

1. Greater inhibition at the junction of the paper strips indicates **synergy** (pictured alongside): The applied antibiotics work together to produce an effect more potent than if each antibiotic were applied singly.
2. No inhibition at this junction indicates an **additive effect**: The potency of an antibiotic combination is roughly equal to the combined potencies of each antibiotic singly.
3. Lesser inhibition at this junction than expected indicates **antagonism**: The potency of the combination is less than the combined potencies of each antibiotic taken separately.

Infobox 11.1

Understanding a drug's mechanism of action is not necessarily a straightforward process, even with today's technologies and techniques. Experiments in the

1930s and 40s to elucidate the mechanism of action of sulfa drugs were treading new ground, and therefore mistakes were only expected. An erroneous view of sulfanilamide's mechanism of action existed in the literature during this time.

Initially, it was believed that sulfanilamide acts as a **bacterial catalase inhibitor**. In 1938, Arthur Locke et al. [7, 8] argued that degradation products of sulfanilamide (such as hydroxylamine and its structural analogues) acted as a bacterial catalase inhibitor. Once inhibited, it was claimed that catalase would no longer eliminate peroxide in and around the bacterial cell, causing it to die of oxidative stress.

Immediately after Locke's publication, at least 50 other articles were published between the years 1938 and 1940, all allegedly verifying sulfanilamide's anti-catalase activity.

## SPECIAL ARTICLES

### ANTI-CATALASE AND THE MECHANISM OF SULFANILAMIDE ACTION

HEALTHY, normal rabbits fed sulfanilamide in adequate dosage survive intradermal infection with type I pneumococcus in greater number than rabbits not so benefited.[1] Blood taken from the rabbit during the period of conferred increase in capacity for resistance has a comparably increased capacity for retarding proliferation of type I pneumococcus *in vitro*.[2] The increase is, possibly, accomplished in an indirect way: the actual checking agent being, not sulfanilamide itself, but hydrogen peroxide.

1 A. Locke, R. B. Locke, R. J. Bragdon and R. R. Mellon, SCIENCE, 86: 228, 1937.
2 A. Locke, E. R. Main and R. R. Mellon, *in preparation*.

The pneumococcus and the hemolytic streptococcus have the property of being able to produce peroxide without, at the same time, being able to prevent peroxide accumulation.[3] Both are sensitive to peroxide injury and depend for peroxide elimination on catalase borrowed from the medium supporting growth. Catalases decompose peroxide and permit growth so long as they remain efficient. They are inactivated by hydroxylamine[4] and by substances related to hydroxylamine in structure or properties.[5, 6]

3 J. W. McLeod and J. Gordon, *Jour. Path. Bact.*, 26: 326, 1923.
4 H. Blaschko, *Biochem. Jour.*, 29: 2302, 1935.
5 D. Keilin and E. F. Hartree, *Nature*, 134: 933, 1934.
6 M. G. Sevag and L. Maiweg, *Biochem. Ztschr.*, 288: 41, 1936.

### THE GERM-KILLING EFFECTIVENESS OF SULFANILAMIDE

**Drs. Mellon and Shinn reported that they had changed the location of one of the chemical units in the complex sulfanilamide molecule and "preformed" it as the germs themselves might do. They left intact the part which the organisms convert into the anti-catalase and, at the same time, moved the new preformed part of the molecule so that much greater stability against the human blood is obtained.**

**So far the results have been only partially successful in this attempt to make a stable "preformed" anti-catalase, but the report states that "These findings . . . lead to the hope that it may be possible to produce prechanged sulfonamide drugs capable of reaching the infecting bacteria."—ROBERT D. POTTER.**

An incorrect understanding of a drug's mechanism of action will lead to incorrect approaches toward that drug's optimization.

Ralph R. Mellon and L.E. Shinn, for example, attempted to optimize sulfanilamide's in vivo stability by chemically altering the molecule but were very careful to **leave intact** the part which **"organisms converted into anti-catalase"** [9], which in hindsight we know does not exist.

As of 1940, their efforts were reported to have been met with "only partial success." Again in hindsight, it is safe to assume their efforts eventually ended in failure.

## THE RELATION OF *p*-AMINOBENZOIC ACID TO THE MECHANISM OF THE ACTION OF SULPHANILAMIDE.

D. D. WOODS.*

Received for publication February 23, 1940.

**A large number of substances known to be associated with bacterial metabolism were tested to determine whether they had an antagonistic relation to sulphanilamide akin to that of –SH and Hg but without conclusive results. While this work was in progress, Stamp (1939), working on a similar hypothesis, found that extracts of streptococci were able to antagonize the action of sulphanilamide and later, while the present paper was actually in preparation, Green (1940) obtained a preparation from *Brucella abortus*. Following Stamp's procedure it was found that yeast extracts contained a substance which, like that of Stamp and Green, reversed the inhibitory action of sulphanilamide. The chemical properties of this substance and its behaviour in growth tests indicated that it might be chemically related to sulphanilamide itself. As a result of this suggestion *p*-aminobenzoic acid was tested and found to have high anti-sulphanilamide activity. A preliminary report of this work has already been given (Woods and Fildes, 1940). The bearing of these results on the possible mode of action of the drug is discussed.**

In 1940 the scientific consensus regarding this topic changed after seminal work published by D.D. Woods described the ability of **yeast extracts to antagonize the action of sulfanilamide** [10]. After meticulous experimentation, Woods isolated **para-amino benzoic acid** (PABA) as the source of this antagonism, leading to our current consensus on the mechanism of action of sulfa drugs.

By 1943, the consensus largely shifted in Woods' favor [11] for several reasons including (but not limited to) the following:

1. Some catalase-negative bacteria displayed sensitivity toward sulfa drugs. Sulfanilamide should not be able to inhibit a strain that does not possess its theoretical target.
2. Organisms normally resistant to peroxide were inhibited by sulfa drugs.
3. Certain anaerobes were inhibited by sulfa drugs. This should not have been theoretically possible since sulfa drugs acted in the absence of conditions necessary for the generation of peroxide.
4. PABA could not inhibit the antimicrobial activity of alleged breakdown products of sulfanilamide.

## 11.4 Resistance Mechanisms

Sulfa drug and trimethoprim resistance can evolve through multiple mechanisms [12]:

1. Mutations on the genes encoding DHPS and DHFR. A **single amino acid substitution** on DHPS [13] or DHFR [14] is sufficient for conferring sulfamethoxazole or trimethoprim resistance, respectively. However clinical isolates usually possess multiple such substitutions.
2. **Overexpression of DHFR**, typically several hundred fold, to offer more targets than there are intracellular trimethoprim molecules [15]. Mutations in the promoter, mutations leading to an optimal ribosome-binding site, and codon optimization within the gene, were credited for this effect.
3. Low-level trimethoprim resistance can develop through the **removal of the ability to methylate nucleotides UMP into TMP** (methionine cycle, Fig. 11.5) via deletion mutations. While this makes the pathogen dependent on an external source of thymine, it eliminates the necessity to constantly regenerate THF from DHF using DHFR (thymidylate cycle, Fig. 11.5), which of course is trimethoprim's target.
4. **Chromosomal recombination** that incorporates a new DHPS gene from a distantly related species. One study [16] reported that the DHPS genes of sulfa-resistant *N. meningitidis* were *10% different* compared to those of sulfa-sensitive **N. meningitidis**. Such a large difference cannot arise from point mutations during human lifetimes.
5. **Efflux pumps**; read Sect. 3.4.3 for more details.

## 11.5 Problems

**Problem 11.1**

1. Will an excess of para-aminobenzoic acid in the culture media reduce the efficacy of sulfamethoxazole? Why or why not?
2. Will an excess of para-aminobenzoic acid in the culture media reduce the efficacy of trimethoprim? Why or why not?
3. If you answered "no" for 2, what small molecule should be added to the culture media to reduce the efficacy of trimethoprim?

**Problem 11.2**

Your guide has created an experimental antimetabolite by covalently linking together trimethoprim and sulfamethoxazole. He expects this construct (trizole-Ω) to possess both anti-DHFR and anti-DHPS activity but would like you to experimentally confirm. It is entirely possible that one or both antibiotics has been inactivated by the fusion. Design a set of NADPH-based colorimetric experiments to determine whether trizole-Ω possesses:

1. No anti-DHFR and no anti-DHPS activity
2. Anti-DHFR activity only
3. Anti-DHPS activity only
4. Both anti-DHFR and anti-DHPS activity

You also have at hand four plasmids for sensitive DHFR, sensitive DHPS, resistant DHFR, and resistant DHPS. List all the ingredients in your initial reaction mix for every experiment.

**Problem 11.3**

An experimental antibiotic inhibits thymidylate synthase: the enzyme that converts UMP into TMP. Testing of the antibiotic has progressed to the in vivo stage and is currently being tested against sensitive *E. coli* in a mouse model of peritonitis. Do you expect it to display synergy, an additive effect, or antagonism when coadministered alongside trimethoprim in this mouse model? Explain.

**Problem 11.4**

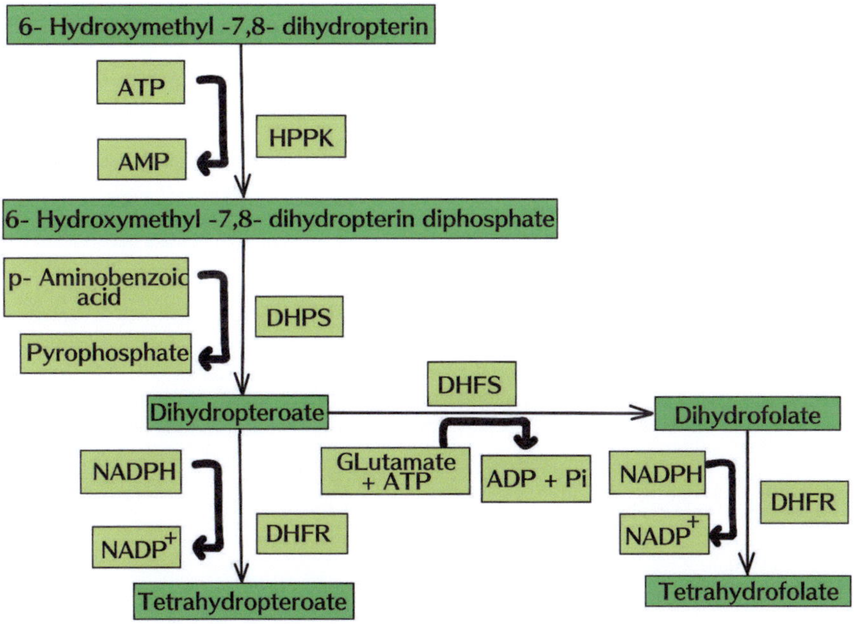


DHFR is also capable of catalyzing the NADPH-mediated reduction of dihydropteroate to tetrahydropteroate. Given this expanded folate pathway, is it

possible to use one or more simple NADPH-based colorimetric assays to test the efficacy of potential DHFS inhibitors? Yes or no?
If yes, describe how you would perform such a colorimetric assay.
If no, suggest an alternate experiment to test the efficacy of potential DHFS inhibitors.

## References


1. Brownlee G (1949) The sulphonamides and allied compounds. Nature 163(4148):662–662
2. Trefouel J, Nitti F, Bovet D (1935) Activité du p-aminophénylsulfonamide sur les infections streptococciques expérimentales de la souris et du lapin. CR Soc Biol (Paris) 120:756–758
3. Wainwright M, Kristiansen JE (2011) On the 75th anniversary of prontosil. Dyes Pigments 88(3):231–234
4. Ballentine C (1981) Sulfanilamide disaster. FDA Consumer Mag, 5
5. Kao SCH, Phan VH, Clarke SJ (2010) Predictive markers for haematological toxicity of pemetrexed. Current Drug Targets 11(1):48–57
6. Fernley RT, Iliades P, Macreadie I (2007) A rapid assay for dihydropteroate synthase activity suitable for identification of inhibitors. Analytic Biochem 360(2):227–234
7. Locke A, Main ER, Mellon RR (1938) Anti-catalase and the mechanism of sulfanilamide action. Science 88(2296):620–621
8. Shinn LE, Main ER, Mellon RR (1938) Anticatalase activity of sulfanilamide and related compounds. ii. relation to growth inhibition in pneumococcus. Proc Soc Exp Biol Med 39(3):591–594
9. Potter RD (1940) The germ-killing effectiveness of sulfanilamide. Science 91(2363):12–14
10. Woods DD (1940) The relation of p-aminobenzoic acid to the mechanism of the action of sulphanilamide. Br J Exp Pathol 21(2):74
11. Henry RJ (1943) The mode of action of sulfonamides. Bacteriol Rev 7(4):198
12. Huovinen P, Sundström L, Swedberg G, Sköld O (1995) Trimethoprim and sulfonamide resistance. Antimicrobial Agents Chemotherapy 39(2):279–289
13. Iliades P, Meshnick SR, Macreadie IG (2004) Dihydropteroate synthase mutations in pneumocystis jiroveci can affect sulfamethoxazole resistance in a Saccharomyces cerevisiae model. Antimicrobial Agents Chemotherapy 48(7):2617–2623
14. Maskell JP, Sefton AM, Hall LMC (2001) Multiple mutations modulate the function of dihydrofolate reductase in trimethoprim-resistant streptococcus pneumoniae. Antimicrobial Agents Chemotherapy 45(4):1104–1108
15. Flensburg J, Sköld O (1987) Massive overproduction of dihydrofolate reductase in bacteria as a response to the use of trimethoprim. Eur J Biochem 162(3):473–476
16. Rådström P, Fermer C, Kristiansen BE, Jenkins A, Sköld O, Swedberg G (1992) Transformational exchanges in the dihydropteroate synthase gene of Neisseria meningitidis: a novel mechanism for acquisition of sulfonamide resistance. J Bacteriol 174(20):6386–6393

# Mycolic Acid Inhibitors

# 12

Pampi Chakraborty

**Abstract**

Tuberculosis, caused by *Mycobacterium tuberculosis*, infects 10 million people annually while causing 1.5 million annual deaths. *M. tuberculosis* possesses a cell wall composed of mycolic acids that are impervious to most drugs. Isoniazid and ethambutol are two mycolic acid inhibitors effective against sensitive strains of *M. tuberculosis*. For isoniazid, mycolic acid inhibition can be assayed using $^{14}$C-labeled n-fatty acids that act as mycolic acid precursors, following the extraction of products and visualization using thin-layer chromatography. Ethambutol inhibits the enzyme arabinosyl transferase, which are required for cell wall assembly. This can be visualized using by tracing the uptake and metabolism of $^{14}$C-labeled glucose into the mycolic-acid-containing cell wall. Mutations within the KatG and InhA genes are responsible for isoniazid resistance. Mutations within the embCAB operon are responsible for ethambutol resistance.

**Keywords**

Tuberculosis · Isoniazid · Ethambutol · Drug resistance

According to the World Health Organization, tuberculosis is currently the biggest cause of mortality among all infectious illnesses globally (WHO). Despite the fact that tuberculosis (TB) is preventable and treatable, 10 million people get the illness annually, and 1.5 million people pass away from it. *Mycobacterium tuberculosis* (MTB), the primary culprit, is currently a major cause of antimicrobial medication

P. Chakraborty (✉)
Department of Microbiology, St. Xavier's College, Mumbai, India
e-mail: pampi.chakraborty@xaviers.edu

© The Editor(s) (if applicable) and The Author(s), under exclusive license to Springer Nature Singapore Pte Ltd. 2024
D. Nagarajan (ed.), *Antibiotics and Their Mechanisms of Action*,
https://doi.org/10.1007/978-981-97-6851-6_12

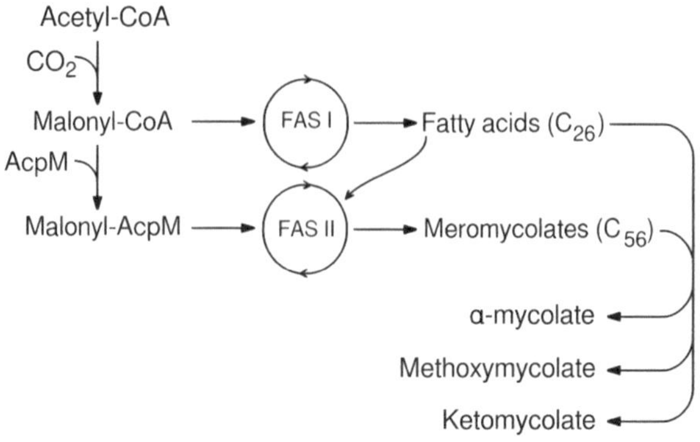


**Fig. 12.1** A simplified representation of **mycolic acid biosynthesis pathways**. A more detailed representation has been compiled by Marrakchi et al. [1]

resistance. *M. tuberculosis* possesses a cell wall composed of mycolic acids that is extremely difficult to penetrate for most antibiotics (Fig. 12.1). The illness has become uncontrollable due to the advent of multidrug-resistant (MDR) and extreme drug-resistant (XDR) TB strains, as well as the failure of the traditional BCG vaccination. For those with HIV, TB seems to be the leading cause of mortality. During the course of therapy for drug-susceptible MTB infection, a combination of four drugs is prescribed, known as first-line drugs. **Isoniazid**, **Rifampicin**, **Pyrazinamide**, and **Ethambutol** are together used for the first 6–9 months in the initial treatment of this disease.

Rifampicin is an RNA polymerase inhibitor and has been discussed in Chap. 7. Pyrazinamide's mechanism of action is currently unknown. This chapter will therefore focus on the mechanisms of action of the other two first-line drugs against TB: isoniazid and ethambutol, both of which are **mycolic acid inhibitors** [1].

Treatment of patients with MDR or XDR tuberculosis involves second-line drugs or reserve drugs like kanamycin, cycloserine, capreomycin, and norfloxacin, which are toxic as well as very expensive.

## 12.1 Isoniazid

**Hans Meyer** and **Josef Mally** from Charles University (Germany) first synthesized isoniazid in 1912 as part of their doctoral study, without knowing the immense potential of the compound for treating TB. In 1951, two groups of scientists from Germany and the Unites States independently demonstrated that isoniazid had a high degree of anti-TB activity. Over the years, isoniazid has proven highly effective, specific, and well-tolerated. The key to the compound's effectiveness turned out to be a pyridine ring in place of a benzene ring (Fig. 12.2).

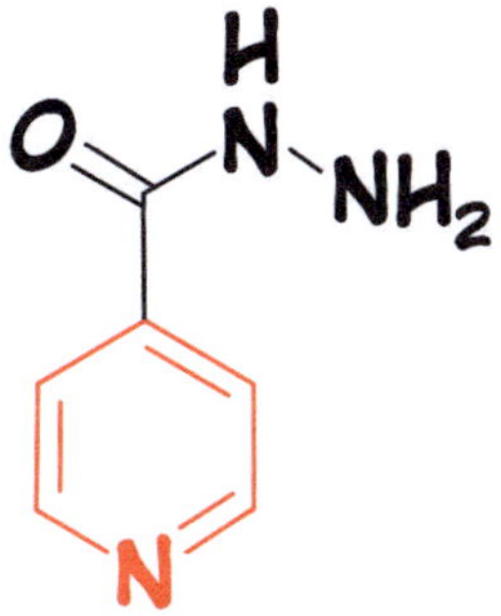


**Fig. 12.2** **The structure of isoniazid**. The pyridine ring is highlighted in red

### 12.1.1 Mechanism of Action

Isoniazid's mechanism of action is complex and is still under study. However, isoniazid ultimately inhibits the synthesis of mycolic acids and their incorporation into the cell wall.

Isoniazid acts as a prodrug, inhibiting bacterial cell wall synthesis following activation by the bacterial catalase–peroxidase enzyme KatG. It induces a variety of radicals, specially the isonicotinic acyl radical which spontaneously couples with NADH to form nicotinyl-NAD adducts that inhibit the production of the mycolic (cell wall component) acids by binding enoyl–acyl carrier protein reductase InhA. This reductase is responsible for the enoyl-AcpM substrate production for fatty acid synthesis. Therefore, INH can block the mycolic acid synthesis, part of bacterial cell wall component of rapidly dividing MTB. It is a bacteriostatic for latent or very slow growing MTB. TB bacilli are susceptible to 0.1–1 μg/mL concentration of INH in several in vitro studies.

To determine the effect of isoniazid on the synthesis of mycolic acid or on its incorporation into the wall, a simple experiment can be performed. *M. tuberculosis* can be exposed to $^{14}$C-labeled n-fatty acids that act as mycolic acid precursors in the growth media. Following growth, apolar cellular contents can be extracted and run on a thin-layer chromatography (TLC) plate. The ratio of fatty acids to mycolic acids on the TLC plate can be determined using a simple radioassay (Fig. 12.3):

1. The untreated control is expected to have incorporated some radiolabelled n-fatty acids into mycolic acids. A spot corresponding to the original n-fatty acid as well as spots corresponding to newly synthesized mycolic acids is expected.
2. The isoniazid-treated culture is expected to synthesize no mycolic acids. Therefore only spots corresponding to the original n-fatty acids will be observed.

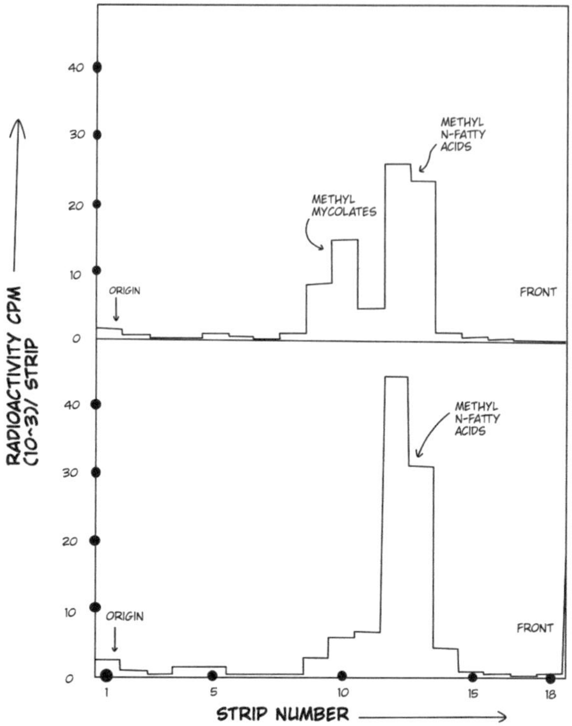


**Fig. 12.3 Isoniazid inhibits the formation of mycolic acids in *M. tuberculosis*. (a)** Untreated cultures displaying the synthesis of mycolic acids from $^{14}C$-labeled n-fatty acids. Both types of molecules were separated and quantified on a TLC plate. **(b)** A culture treated with isoniazid displaying no newly synthesized mycolic acids on a TLC plate

### 12.1.2 Isoniazid Resistance Mechanisms

Gene mutations within KatG and InhA were observed for isoniazid-resistant organisms. For this reason, the drug is employed in combination with other antimycobacterial agents (especially ethambutol or rifampicin) to reduce the emergence of resistant tubercle bacilli.

## 12.2 Ethambutol

Ethambutol (Fig. 12.4) is a synthetic, water-soluble, heat-stable drug against many typical and "atypical" strains of *M. tuberculosis* in the concentration range 1–5 μg/mL. It was first discovered at Lederle Laboratories of American Cynamid in

**Fig. 12.4 Structure of ethambutol**

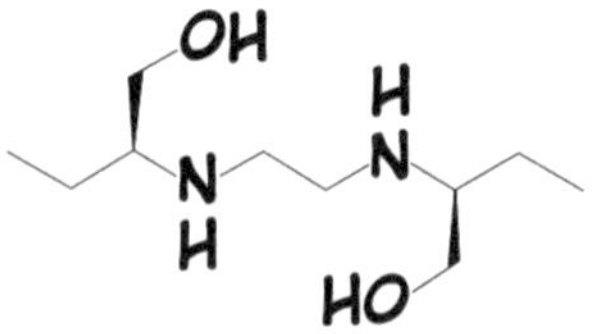

1961. The drug is remarkably stereospecific. The dextro form of the drug is 12 times more active than the meso form, whereas the levo form is entirely inactive.

### 12.2.1 Mechanism of Action

Ethambutol is also a mycobacterial mycolic acid synthesis inhibitor which inhibits the enzyme arabinosyl transferase. The enzyme polymerizes arabinose to arabinan and arabinogalactan which is a cell wall component of MTB. Early experiments confirmed the immediate accumulation of the major intermediates of mycolic acid synthesis for the cell wall.

The in vivo synthesis of arabinogalactan and arabinomannan can be assayed in the presence or absence of Ethambutol [2]. A *Mycobacterium smegmatis* broth culture is kept with 1 μCi of uniformly labelled $^{14}$C-glucose at 37°C for the desired time in two fractions. After 2.5 minutes, Ethambutol is added to the test fraction. The cells are killed and harvested by centrifugation after desired time of drug exposure / control. The cell pellet is processed for arabinogalactan and arabinomannan fraction (55 to 85% ethanol-insoluble fraction) after discarding the glucan from each sample. This residue is washed three times with ethanol and is finally dissolved in water. A portion of this solution is taken for radioactivity determination. Figure 12.5 represents the radioactive counts per sample. It is very evident from the result that Ethambutol has reduced the total content of arabinogalactan and arabinomannan in treated samples compared to untreated.

It is therefore clear that ethambutol is able to inhibit the conversion of labelled glucose into arabinose in oligosaccharides present on *M. smegmatis* cell wall.

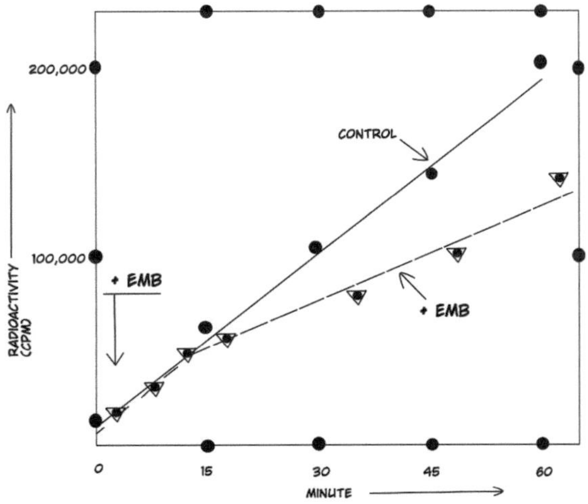


**Fig. 12.5** **Effect of ethambutol** (EMB) on the time course of synthesis of **arabinomannan and arabinogalactan** in cells of ethambutol-susceptible M. smegmatis. The assay measured the incorporation of label from [14C]glucose into the 55 to 85% ethanol-insoluble fraction which represents mycolic acid. The drug (3μg/ml) was added to the culture at 2.5 min (arrow)

### 12.2.2 Ethambutol Resistance Mechanisms

Ethambutol resistance can develop via mutations in the embCAB operon, containing genes embC,A,B. This cluster contains genes responsible for mycobacterial **arabinosyl transferases** [3].

## 12.3 Problems

**Problem 12.1**

Two treatment regimens are proposed for eliminating a sensitive strain of tuberculosis from a patient:

1. Isoniazid for 1 week, ethambutol for 1 week, pyrazinamide for 1 week, rifampicin for 1 week
2. Isoniazid, ethambutol, pyrazinamide, rifampicin, all administered simultaneously for 1 week

Which treatment regimen is better? Why?

**Problem 12.2**

You have isolated the gene coding for arabinosyl transferase and synthesized it into a plasmid. You have added a 6x HIS-tag to the N-terminal and purified the protein using NiNTA chromatography. Now that you have the enzyme at hand, design an experiment to confirm that your enzyme polymerizes arabinan in vitro. Design a similar experiment to confirm that ethambutol inhibits arabinosyl transferase.

**Problem 12.3**

Design an experiment to confirm the mechanism of isoniazid without using isotopes (radioactive or otherwise).

## References

1. Marrakchi H, Lanéelle M-A, Daffé M (2014) Mycolic acids: structures, biosynthesis, and beyond. Chem Biol 21(1):67–85
2. Takayama K, Kilburn JO (1989) Inhibition of synthesis of arabinogalactan by ethambutol in Mycobacterium smegmatis. Antimicrobial Agents Chemotherapy 33(9):1493–1499
3. Telenti A, Philipp WJ, Sreevatsan S, Bernasconi C, Stockbauer KE, Wieles B, Musser JM, Jacobs WR (1997) The emb operon, a gene cluster of Mycobacterium tuberculosis involved in resistance to ethambutol. Nature Med 3(5):567–570

# Other Antimicrobial Agents 13

Aparna Shetye and Deepesh Nagarajan

**Abstract**

Over 100 different antibiotics have been approved for clinical use. This number does not include the list of approved antiviral, antifungal, and antiprotozoal agents. Existing antivirals are predominantly used against the influenza and HIV viruses. It is difficult to discover antivirals due to the viral ability to hijack host metabolic machinery, the difficulty in culturing viruses, and their high mutation rates. Antifungal agents predominantly target fungal cell wall synthesis as well as ergosterol synthesis. Antiprotozoals are used to treat amoebiasis, leishmaniasis, malaria, and trypanosomiasis. A brief summary of important drugs in these classes is provided in the chapter.

**Keywords**

Antivirals · Antifungals · Antiprotozoals

Over 100 different antibiotics have been approved for clinical use, and this number does not include all other anti-infectious agents. It would be an arduous task to describe every single one of these drugs in detail.

A. Shetye (✉)
Department of Microbiology, St. Xavier's College, Mumbai, India
e-mail: aparna.talekar@xaviers.edu

D. Nagarajan
Department of Microbiology, St. Xavier's College, Mumbai, India

Department of Biotechnology, M.S. Ramaiah University of Applied Sciences, Bangalore, India
e-mail: deepeshn.bt.ls@msruas.ac.in; deepesh.nagarajan@xaviers.edu

© The Editor(s) (if applicable) and The Author(s), under exclusive license to Springer Nature Singapore Pte Ltd. 2024

D. Nagarajan (ed.), *Antibiotics and Their Mechanisms of Action*,
https://doi.org/10.1007/978-981-97-6851-6_13

This book has described select antibiotics and their mechanisms of action. Understanding the workings of the antibiotics described here should equip the reader with the skills needed to study any other antibiotic, or perhaps even experimentally decipher a new antibiotic's mechanism of action.

This chapter presents a brief summary of anti-infectious agents not covered in this book. At least **90 antiviral** [1], **23 antifungal** [1], and **16 antiprotozoal** agents [2] have been approved for clinical use. The reader is encouraged to explore these drugs in more detail than provided here.

## 13.1 Antiviral Agents

**Idoxuridine**, the first antiviral agent described, was developed against **Herpesviruses**. This development occurred in 1963, approximately half a century after the description of the first antibiotic. Currently, a little over 90 antivirals are approved for use in humans. These are useful against roughly around 10 viral infections. The slow pace of antiviral drug discovery highlights the differences infection cycles of viruses and other pathogens. Some of the reasons for this slow pace and a limited number of infections they target also lie in workings of the pharmaceutical industry and the growing costs of clinical trials (see Sect. 1.3.3).

Why do we have so few antivirals at our disposal?

1. Most viruses lack enzymes and any **machinery needed for their replication**. All use the protein synthesis machinery of the host and only some carry enzymes needed for replication of their nucleic acid. Therefore it is difficult to target viral replication and expression processes since they are shared with the host cells. Most antivirals thus also display more toxicity in general than agents that inhibit other pathogens. Nevertheless, some viral processes can be targeted as outlined later.
2. **Cultivation of viruses** is considerably more difficult that other pathogens. Many viruses lack a suitable cell culture system or animal model. Testing of antivirals against these is obviously difficult.
3. Many viral diseases are acute and have **very short onset periods**. It is thus often difficult to start therapy before the peak of the disease cycle is reached.
4. Unlike antibiotics, the concept of "broad spectrum" does not really exist among antivirals. Most antivirals target one or **at the most 2–3-related viruses**. Most viruses use completely different infection cycles and thus selectivity is usually the norm.
5. Many viruses, especially RNA viruses, have a **high mutation rate** which translates into faster emergence of resistance. Many drugs used in the past such as amantadine against Influenza and enfuvirtide against HIV showed appearance of resistant mutants within few years of clinical use. Antivirals thus have to be very effective to prevent resistance development.

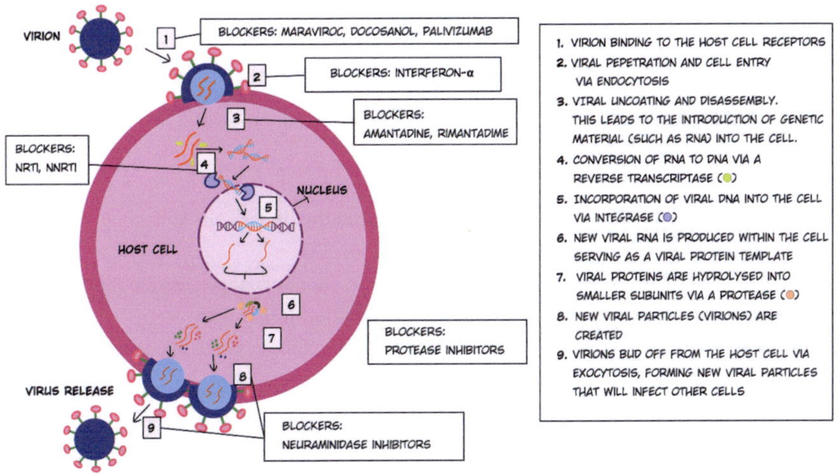


**Fig. 13.1** **The generalized viral life cycle**, along with agents that target every step of the cycle. Table 13.1 tabulates all the agents illustrated here

6. Diagnostic procedures are lacking or not commonplace for many viral infections. This together with the lack of broad antivirals means that many viral diseases cannot be treated in a timely manner.

The generalized viral infection cycle and drug targets along with a few important antiviral agents are illustrated in Fig. 13.1 and listed in Table 13.1. However this is not an exhaustive list.

## 13.2 Antifungal Agents

Fungal infections in humans range from the annoying but mundane conditions like onychomycosis (fungal infection of the nail) and athletes foot to life-threatening conditions like cryptococcal meningitis. Due to the diverse range of diseases caused by fungi, it is clinically prudent to classify them into superficial, subcutaneous, and systemic mycoses. Fungal infections are generally harder to treat compared to bacterial infections because:

1. Unlike bacteria, fungi are **eukaryotes**. Their structure and metabolic machinery more closely resemble their human hosts than bacteria and are therefore harder to target selectively using an antibiotic.
2. Fungi have **innate detoxification systems** that eliminate antifungals. Antifungal treatment therefore required the repeated and prolonged administration of anti-fungal agents.

**Table 13.1 Select antivirals and their mechanisms of action**, as illustrated in Fig. 13.1. Important terminology: **Reverse transcriptase**: an enzyme that reverse-transcribes viral RNA to DNA. **NRTIs**: Nucleoside/nucleotide reverse transcriptase inhibitors. **NNRTIs**: Non-nucleoside/nucleotide reverse transcriptase inhibitors. **Viral protease**: HIV viral proteins are encoded within a single gene. The single polypeptide chain translated from this gene is cleaved into multiple proteins using a viral protease

| Antiviral | Mechanism of action |
|---|---|
| Docosanol, maraviroc, palivizumab | **Attachment inhibitor**: Blocks virion binding to the host cell receptor |
| Interferon-$\alpha$ (natural cytokine) enfuvirtide | **Fusion inhibitor**: Blocks viral penetration into the host cell via endocytosis |
| Amantadine, rimantadine | **Uncoating inhibitor** Blocks virion uncoating and disassembly within the host cell |
| **Antiretroviral drugs** | |
| NRTI: zidovudine, lamivudine | Reverse transcriptase inhibitors |
| NNRTI: efavirenz, nevirapine | Reverse transcriptase inhibitors |
| Viral protease inhibitors | Inhibit viral protease. |
| Zanamivir, oseltamivir | **Neuraminidase inhibitors** Block the formation of new virions via budding / exocytosis |

A healthy human with good personal hygiene has little to fear from pathogenic fungi. Most deaths due to mycosis occur in severely immunocompromised patients (suffering from AIDS, being administered immunosuppressants, or with other comorbidities).

A list of antifungal agents is provided in Table 13.2. It is by no means exhaustive.

**Ergosterol** (Fig. 13.2) is a critical component of fungal cell membranes that is absent in human cell membranes. Its biochemical synthesis pathways therefore offer tempting drug targets. Several unrelated antifungals inhibit ergosterols:

1. The **Triazoles**: These antifungals bind to and inhibit fungal cytochrome P-450, thereby interrupting the conversion of lanosterol to ergosterol. This leads to the disruption of fungal cell membranes.
2. **Terbinafine** and **naftifine** inhibit squalene epoxidase. This enzyme converts qualene into 2,3(S)-oxidosqualene and is a critical step in the fungal cholesterol and ergosterol biosynthesis pathways.

## 13.3 Antiprotozoal Agents

Protozoans cause a diverse range of diseases which can be categorized as follows:

1. **Amoebiasis**: Intestinal infections that cause diarrhea. Treated using metronidazole, tinidazole, and diloxanide furoate.

**Table 13.2** Select antifungals and their mechanisms of action

| Antifungal | Mechanism of action |
|---|---|
| **Echinocandins** | |
| Caspofungin, micafungin, anidulafungin | Inhibits fungal cell wall synthesis |
| **Triazoles** | |
| Fluconazole, itraconazole<br>Voriconazole, Posaconazole | Inhibits ergosterol synthesis |
| Terbinafine, naftifine | Inhibits ergosterol synthesis |
| Amphotericin-B, Nystatin | Binds to fungal cell membrane |
| 5-flucytosine | Inhibits fungal of DNA/RNA synthesis |
| Griseofulvin | Disrupts the fungal mitotic spindle |

**Fig. 13.2** The structure of ergosterol

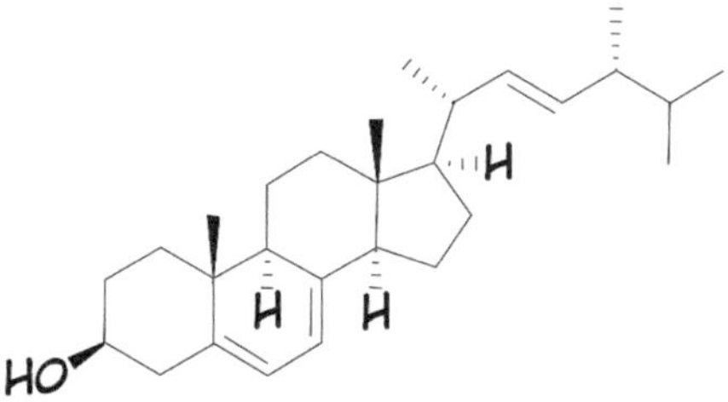


2. **Leishmaniasis**: A neglected tropical disease spread through the bite of phlebotomine sandflies. Typically it causes ulcers on the skin, mouth, and nose. Treated using sodium stibogluconate and amphotericin B.
3. **Malaria**: Caused by *Plasmodium spps* and spread through the bite of mosquitoes. Treated using quinine (obsolete), chloroquine, mefloquine, atovaquone, tetracycline, and primaquine.
4. **Trypanosomiasis**: Sleeping sickness caused by *Trypanosoma brucei*. Treated using melarsoprol, pentamidine, eflornithine, nifurtimox, benznidazole.
5. **Other diseases**: Toxoplasmosis, microsporidiosis, trichomoniasis.

Like fungi, protozoans are eukaryotes and are therefore harder to develop drugs against. Protozoans also have complex life cycles and diverse biochemistry, making treatment against one protozoan ineffective against another. A list of antiprotozoal agents and their mechanisms of action is given in Table 13.3. This list is by no means exhaustive.

It should be noted that antifungal agents like amphotericin B and antibacterial agents like tetracycline also possess antiprotozoal activity. Antibiotics are now known to possess multiple mechanisms of action. If a single antibiotic can act on multiple drug targets within a single pathogen, it is possible that some could act on drug targets from pathogens in different kingdoms of life as well.

**Table 13.3** Select antiprotozoals and their mechanisms of action

| Antiprotozoal | Mechanism of action |
|---|---|
| Metronidazole, tinidazole | Interacts with DNA. Causes the loss of DNA helicity, strand breakage |
| Sodium stibogluconate | Unknown, possibly inhibits ATP formation |
| diloxanide furoate | Unknown |
| Quinine, chloroquine | Inhibits nucleic acid synthesis, protein synthesis, and glycolysis in *Plasmodium spps* |
| | Also binds with hemozoin in parasitized erythrocytes |
| Mefloquine | Unknown, possibly targets the 80S protozoal ribosome, preventing protein synthesis |
| Atovaquone | Inhibits electron transport |
| Melarsoprol | Binds to pyruvate kinase and inhibits glycolysis |
| Pentamidine | Unknown, possibly inhibits the synthesis of DNA, RNA, phospholipids, and proteins |
| Eflornithine | Ornithine decarboxylase inhibitor. Inhibits polyamine synthesis |
| Nifurtimox | Unknown. Possibly activates nitroreductase enzymes |
| Benznidazole | Unknown, possibly inhibits the synthesis of DNA, RNA, and proteins |

## References

1. De Clercq E, Li G (2016) Approved antiviral drugs over the past 50 years. Clin Microbiol Rev 29(3):695–747
2. Thurston S, Hite GL, Petry AN, Ray SD (2015) Antiprotozoal drugs. Side Effects Drugs Annual 37:321–327

# 14 Antibiotic Pharmacology and Biopharmaceutics

Subhrojyoti Ghosh, Varshaa Arer, and Debasish Kar

**Abstract**

Pharmacology is the branch of medicine pertaining to the uses, effects, and modes of action of drugs. Biopharmaceutics explores the association between the characteristics and magnitude of biological effects observed in both animals and humans. This chapter discusses pharmacological drug target systems, biopharmaceutics classification systems, and the pharmaceutics of all antibiotics previously covered in this book, from penicillin to mycolic acid inhibitors. Case studies are also provided where appropriate.

**Keywords**

Pharmacology · Biopharmaceutics · Pharmaceutics · ADME

## 14.1 Introduction

The discipline of pharmacology has a rich historical background, tracing its origin back to ancient civilizations and herblore [1]. Hippocrates, credited as founder of medicine, placed a significant value on empirical knowledge, rather than mystical beliefs, within the field [2]. In the 1st century AD, the Greek physician Dioscorides composed *De Materia Medica*, documenting the properties and applications of

S. Ghosh (✉) · V. Arer
Department of Biotechnology, Indian Institute of Technology, Madras, India
e-mail: bt22m010@smail.iitm.ac.in; 20larp715007@msruas.ac.in

D. Kar
Department of Biotechnology, M.S. Ramaiah University of Applied Sciences, Bangalore, India
e-mail: debasish.bt.ls@msruas.ac.in

© The Editor(s) (if applicable) and The Author(s), under exclusive license to Springer Nature Singapore Pte Ltd. 2024
D. Nagarajan (ed.), *Antibiotics and Their Mechanisms of Action*,
https://doi.org/10.1007/978-981-97-6851-6_14

various medicinal plants [3]. Researchers during the Islamic Golden age played a crucial role in preserving and advancing the field of pharmaceutical knowledge [4]. The establishment of pharmacology as an academic field occurred in the $19^{th}$ century [5] amid a resurgence in the biomedical fields. Early in the $20^{th}$ century, the Food and Drug Administration (FDA) and other regulatory bodies were established, along with the strict guidelines pertaining to the safety and efficacy of drugs [6]. Individuals such as Rudolf Buchheim and Oswald Schmeideberg also played a significant role in the development of pharmaceutical research and education [7] and are considered the founders of modern pharmacology. Today, pharmacology has greatly broadened its scope, encompassing rapidly advancing fields like pharmacogenomics and nanomedical pharmacology, and biopharmaceutics.

The term biopharmaceutics is a recent addition to the field of pharmaceutical science [8]. In its most expansive interpretation, biopharmaceutics can be characterized as the examination of the complex connection between specific physical and chemical attributes of a drug and its dosage forms, along with the resulting biological effects witnessed upon the administration of the drug in diverse forms. This comprehensive definition significantly overlaps with pharmacology and encompasses a wide range of areas, including drug latency [9] and the creation of different salts of an acidic or basic drug with the aim of modifying the biological effects produced by the original drug. Therefore, biopharmaceutics explores the association between the characteristics and magnitude of biological effects observed in both animals and humans, considering various critical factors [10]:

1. Simple **chemical modifications** of drugs, such as forming esters, salts, and complexes
2. Alterations in the physical state, particle size, and surface area of the drug, which influence its availability at **absorption sites**
3. The presence or absence of **adjuvants** within the dosage form and the drug
4. The specific type of **dosage** form used to administer the drug
5. The pharmaceutical processes employed in the **manufacturing** of the dosage form

Fundamentally, biopharmaceutics encompasses the process of drug absorption, playing a pivotal role in the systemic uptake of most drug products. This absorption involves a sequence of rate processes, encompassing the disintegration of the product, dissolution of the drug in an aqueous environment, and permeation across cell membranes into the systemic circulation, ultimately reaching its site of action. Overcoming obstacles like aqueous solubility, stability, permeability, and the first-pass effect is crucial for transporting a drug from its dosage form to its intended site of action. The challenges posed by these factors may vary depending on formulation efforts [9]. When it becomes apparent that a potential drug candidate displays suboptimal biopharmaceutical properties, thoughtful consideration must be given to its developability.

Various mathematical models have been proposed in the literature to estimate oral absorption and bioavailability. One such model, the absorption potential (AP) introduced by Dressman et al. in 1985 [11], has shown quantitative correlations with fraction absorbed and serves as a valuable indicator of the critical limiting physicochemical property for poorly absorbed compounds. However, it is important to note that the AP primarily focuses on the drug's physicochemical properties and cannot be solely relied upon to assess bioavailability [9].

On the contrary, the mathematical models established by Sinko et al. in 1991 have shown robust correlations between in vitro dissolution and in vivo bioavailability [12]. These models highlight three dimensionless numbers: absorption number (An), dissolution number (Dn), and dose number (Do), representing crucial processes associated with membrane permeation, drug dissolution, and dosage, respectively [13]. These parameters can be computed for a new molecule and subsequently employed to predict the extent of drug absorption by referring to contour plots [14]. Nevertheless, it is important to recognize that all these dimensionless numbers are fundamentally connected to two pivotal parameters governing drug absorption: solubility and permeability. In consideration of this, the Biopharmaceutic Drug Classification Scheme (BCS) was introduced by Amidon et al. in 1995 [13]. BCS has become a vital tool for developing effective strategies to enhance the bioavailability of new chemical entities. When facing biopharmaceutic challenges, there are two primary strategies to consider. The first involves formulation efforts aimed at overcoming these hurdles without consuming excessive time and resources. If successful, this approach allows for modifications in drug formulation. The second strategy involves chemical modifications to the structure of the lead compound to address biopharmaceutical obstacles. In the context of the expanding libraries of compounds resulting from combinatorial chemistry and high-throughput screening, major pharmaceutical companies have adopted innovative approaches to select suitable candidates for further development. These approaches consider biopharmaceutic properties such as solubility, permeability, and various physicochemical parameters.

## 14.2 Terms and Definitions

1. **Maximum Serum Concentration** ($C_{max}$): It refers to the highest plasma concentration reached by a drug after administration.
2. **Minimum time for** $C_{max}$ ($t_{max}$): It represents the shortest duration taken for the drug to achieve its peak plasma concentration.
3. **Half-life** ($t_{1/2}$): Elimination half-life is the time needed for the drug concentration to decrease to half of its initial level.
4. **Area Under the Curve (AUC)**: It corresponds to the integral of the concentration-time curve, calculated either after a single dose or in a steady state. These pharmacokinetic parameters are crucial in understanding a drug's behavior within the body, aiding in dosage regimen design and overall therapeutic efficacy assessment.
5. **Bioavailability of a Drug**: Bioavailability pertains to how quickly and to what extent the active moiety (drug or metabolite) enters the systemic circulation,

reaching the site of action. The bioavailability of a drug is predominantly shaped by the characteristics of the dosage form, influenced in part by its design and manufacturing processes.

6. **Bioequivalence of a Drug**: Bioequivalence is a concept within pharmacokinetics (Infobox 14.3) that evaluates the anticipated in vivo biological similarity between two proprietary medication formulations. If two products are deemed bioequivalent, it indicates that, in practical terms, they are anticipated to be identical.

## 14.3 Pharmacological Drug Classification

A substance with a defined chemical structure that induces specific biological effects in a living organism, excluding nutrients or dietary supplements, is termed as a drug. The classification of drugs in pharmacology is complicated due to the lack of universally applicable methodologies. The classification is based on the preferences of chemists, pharmacologists, and healthcare professionals [15]. Nevertheless, drugs may be commonly classified based on four different schemes:

1. **Pharmacological action** Medical professionals have acknowledged the variable medical conditions that they intend to treat. For example:

   - **Analgesics**: These agents are utilized for managing and treating pain. Acetaminophen is an example [16].
   - **Antibiotics**: These interventions target infectious diseases, aiming to prevent progression or facilitate reversal. Vancomycin, for instance, is used in the treatment of colitis [17] (also refer to Chap. 4).
   - **Drugs that target physiological mechanisms**: Modern medicine is sometimes incapable of addressing the fundamental etiology of a disease but is capable of minimizing its impact in an individual. Indapamide, for example, can be used in treatment of hypertension [18].

2. **Mode of action**: Drugs that target a particular biochemical pathway. A biochemical pathway is a series of chemical reactions that take place within a cell or an organism for the purpose of maintaining its regular physiological activity. For example, diabetic ketoacidosis, a disorder of carbohydrate metabolism, is treated with insulin [19] (also refer to Chap. 11).
3. **Molecular targets**: Drugs target a wide range of biomolecules including lipids (refer to Chap. 5), proteins (refer to Chaps. 3, 4, 8), and nucleic acids Chap. 6.
4. **Chemical structure**: Drugs possessing analogous chemical structures typically have comparable pharmacological effects and demonstrate similar mode of actions. For example, penicillin, ampicillin, cefepime, and meropenem are classified as $\beta$-lactams as they all possess a $\beta$-lactam ring, or a derivative thereof (refer to Chap. 3).

**Infobox 14.1**

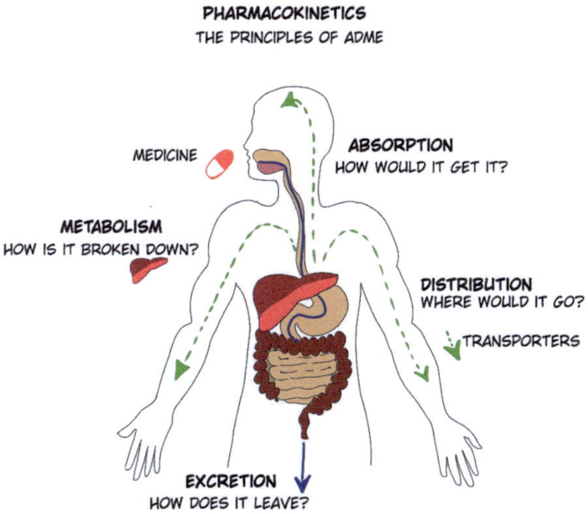


Pharmacokinetics involves studying a drug's journey through the body. This journey can be broken down into four different stages: absorption, distribution, metabolism, and excretion (ADME):

1. **Absorption**: Deals with the drugs immediate journey from its point of administration (oral, intramuscular, intravenous, subcutaneous).
2. **Distribution**: Describes the journey of the drug through the body, usually through the bloodstream. Distribution begins where absorption ends. Distribution ends when the drug reaches its site of action. For antibiotics, this site of action is usually an infected tissue or organ.
3. **Metabolism**: Deals with biochemical processes that break down the drug. Such processes usually occur in the liver and bloodstream.
4. **Excretion**: Deals with the elimination of the drug from the body. Drugs can be excreted via urine, feces, sweat, saliva, tears, bile, and breastmilk.

An ideal drug possesses ideal ADME properties. It should be easily administered and readily absorbed. It should reach the site of action rapidly and in sufficient concentrations. It should possess a high-serum half-life. It should not damage the liver or other organs during metabolism. It should not damage the kidneys or other organs during excretion. Chemical modification techniques attempt to improve a drug's ADME properties to reach these ideals.

## 14.4 Biopharmaceutics Classification System

The biopharmaceutics classification system (BCS) classifies drug substances or APIs based on their solubility and permeability characteristics into four classes. Class I includes drugs with high solubility and high permeability, where the rate-limiting step is typically drug dissolution. Class II consists of drugs with low solubility but high permeability, where in vivo drug dissolution becomes the rate-limiting step for absorption unless at very high doses. Class III drugs have high solubility but low permeability, with permeability being the rate-limiting step for drug absorption, resulting in variable absorption rates. Class IV drugs, characterized by low solubility and permeability, often pose challenges for effective oral administration. The classification, aligned with WHO guidelines, considers parameters such as absorption number, dissolution number, and dose number, offering insights into the key factors influencing bioavailability. Overall, the BCS classification aids in understanding the critical interplay of dissolution, solubility, and permeability in drug absorption. Figure 14.1 illustrates the schematics of BCS.

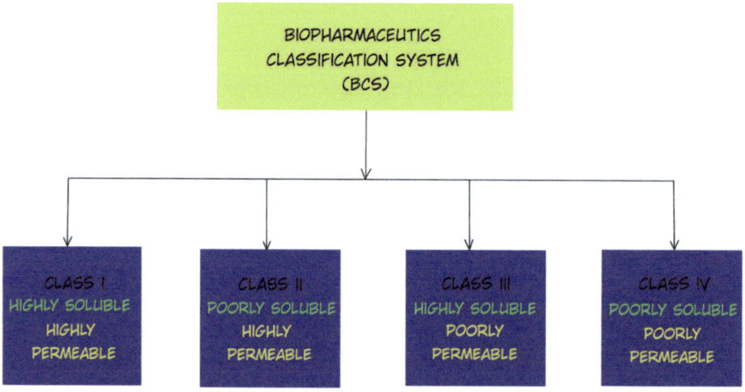


**Fig. 14.1** The **Biopharmaceutics Classification System (BCS)** categorizes drugs into four classes based on solubility and permeability, guiding drug development strategies. This schematic illustrates the key principles of BCS, aiding in the prediction of drug bioavailability for optimized therapeutic outcomes

## 14.5 Biopharmaceutics: Factors Involved

The biopharmaceutics of a drug, particularly its solubility and permeability, are intricately influenced by factors such as molecular structure, aqueous solubility and membrane permeation characteristics, crucial determinants of drug absorption and bioavailability.

### 14.5.1 Solubility

Solubility is a critical factor in drug liberation and absorption, directly influencing a drug's bioavailability [20]. To be absorbed effectively, a drug must be present in the form of an aqueous solution at the absorption site. This principle holds true for various mechanisms of absorption, except for rare cases such as pinocytosis, which primarily applies to fat-soluble compounds like vitamins A, D, E, K, and certain lipids [13]. Insoluble or poorly soluble drugs pose challenges in dissolution and absorption since drug flux across the intestinal membrane depends on the concentration gradient between the apical and basolateral sides of the gastrointestinal lumen [13]. As a result, the aqueous solubility of drugs holds central importance throughout all phases of drug development, from molecular design to pharmaceutical formulation and biopharmaceutics.

The solubility of solid compounds in aqueous media is affected by interactions within the crystal lattice, intermolecular interactions in solution, and entropy changes associated with fusion and dissolution [20]. The observed mole fraction solubility of a solute ($X_w$) is connected to its ideal mole fraction solubility ($X_i$) and the activity coefficient in water ($\gamma_w$). The insolubility of a solute can be influenced by both the crystalline structure and the activity coefficient [20]. Enhancing the solubility of poorly soluble solutes can be achieved through two approaches. One method involves augmenting its ideal solubility through chemical modifications or solid-state manipulations [13]. The second strategy is to reduce its activity coefficient to unity through formulation modifications, such as micellar solubilization, cosolvency, hydrotrophy, and the formation of inclusion complexes [20].

Several drug development examples underscore the importance of solubility [21]. Peptidomimetics, such as HIV protease inhibitors, were initially designed with excellent inhibitory properties but had poor aqueous solubility, high lipophilicity, and other pharmacokinetic challenges [21]. Effective drugs with improved oral bioavailability have been achieved by optimizing physicochemical properties, such as solubility, through chemical modifications. For instance, Vacca et al. (1991) developed hydroxyethylene dipeptide isosteres, which, despite being highly potent and selective HIV protease inhibitors, had limited aqueous solubility and pharmacokinetic profiles [22]. By introducing a basic amine into the compound, they improved solubility and further modifications led to drugs like Indinavir with enhanced aqueous solubility and consistent bioavailability [21].

Similar approaches have been applied in the development of fibrinogen receptor antagonists and other therapeutic compounds, where poor oral activity was attributed to low aqueous solubility. Prodrug strategies have also been employed to enhance aqueous solubility. An increase in solubility does not necessarily guarantee improved bioavailability, as permeability across the gastrointestinal membrane requires lipophilic properties [23]. Therefore, if chemical modification is not feasible, formulation approaches can be used, including the formation of water-soluble salts, pH adjustment, the use of water-miscible cosolvents, surface-active agents, complexing agents, liposomes, and clathrate formation [23].

Cyclodextrins are commonly employed as complexing agents to enhance the solubility of poorly soluble drugs [24]. These complexes have been found to significantly improve dissolution rates and bioavailability for various compounds. For instance, miconazole's solubility increased substantially when complexed with hydroxypropyl—cyclodextrins, leading to improved oral bioavailability in rats and enhanced transdermal diffusivity [24]. Similar positive effects have been observed with other poorly soluble drugs, including hydrocortisone, digitoxin, diazepam, indomethacin, iotraconazole, kynostatin, pilocarpine, cinnarizine, naproxen, and thiabendazole using natural and substituted cyclodextrins [24].

### 14.5.2 Permeability

Permeability, the ability of a molecule to traverse biological membranes, plays a pivotal role in drug pharmacokinetics, impacting processes like absorption, distribution, metabolism, and excretion [25]. Drugs must navigate the transition from lipid biomembranes to aqueous biological fluids during their journey to the biophase. These biomembranes primarily consist of phospholipids, cholesterol, sphingolipids, and glycolipids, all of which exhibit amphipathic properties. To effectively traverse various biomembranes and reach their target sites, drug molecules must strike a balance between their hydrophilic and lipophilic characteristics [25].

The octanol–water partition coefficient (P) is a fundamental property used to assess a compound's lipophilic or hydrophilic nature. It is determined as the ratio of the concentration of the unionized compound in mutually saturated octanol and water. Given that P values can vary across multiple orders of magnitude, the logarithm (log P) is a frequently employed convenience [25]. N-octanol is often chosen as the non-aqueous solvent for such measurements because it closely mimics biological membranes, possessing a saturated alkyl chain, a hydroxyl group for hydrogen bonding, limited water solubility, and a solubility parameter that approximates that of biological membranes [25]. However, the relationship between log P or log D (octanol/water) values and pharmacokinetic parameters doesn't hold for certain drug classes, like peptides, amide-containing drugs, and basic amines [26]. Some basic amines exhibit higher membrane partitioning than expected based on their log D values, mainly because biomembranes can facilitate the partitioning of both neutral and positively charged amine forms [27]. Similarly, peptides' numerous polar functionalities form hydrogen bonds with hydroxyl groups in the aqueous phase, making their log D values less indicative of permeability [27]. Instead, partition coefficients between heptane–ethylene glycol or differences in partition coefficients between octanol buffer and isooctane/cyclohexane buffer (*Delta* log P) are better models for permeability, particularly for peptides and amides [28].

Though no universal rule applies to all drug molecules, within a homologous series of drugs, absorption generally increases with higher lipophilicity up to a certain point, after which it may decline. A log P value between 0 and 3 is usually optimal for passive drug absorption, as values below 0 signify hydrophilicity with good solubility but potential poor permeability, and values far above 3 tend to favor absorption but increase susceptibility to metabolism and biliary clearance [29].

Lipophilicity significantly impacts drug metabolism, as highly lipophilic compounds tend to bind more strongly to enzymes, which can affect their clearance [30]. Predictive methods for log P, despite their limitations, are valuable in the pharmaceutical industry, where experimental measurements can be challenging. These methods generally fall into three categories: fragment constant methods, atomic contribution-based methods, and molecular property-based methods. Examples of drugs that highlight the influence of lipophilicity on oral absorption and subsequent development are evident in the case of renin inhibitors and systemic antifungal agents [31]. Structural modifications based on log P values led to enhanced oral absorption profiles. These cases underscore the importance of lipophilicity in drug discovery and development and its impact on absorption, metabolism, protein binding, and distribution, as well as potential pharmacokinetic drug interactions when administered concomitantly with other drugs [29]. 15.5 Biopharmaceutics of Drug Absorption and Excretion: Absorption is the process through which a drug moves from the site of administration to its site of action [32, 33]. The drug follows a specific route of administration, which can be oral, topical-dermal, or another method, and is typically presented in a specific dosage form, such as tablets, capsules, or a solution [33]. For routes like intravenous therapy, intramuscular injection, or enteral nutrition, absorption is more straightforward and often exhibits near 100% bioavailability with less variability [33]. It's important to note that intravascular administration doesn't involve absorption, and no drug loss occurs [33]. Inhalation is the quickest route for absorption [32]. Understanding and optimizing absorption is a fundamental aspect of drug development and medicinal chemistry because a drug must be absorbed to produce its intended therapeutic effects. Furthermore, adjusting various factors influencing absorption can significantly alter a drug's pharmacokinetic profile.

Biopharmaceutics of drug excretion is a critical aspect of pharmacology that involves the study of the processes by which the body eliminates drugs. The elimination of drugs is primarily mediated through renal excretion, hepatic metabolism, and other pathways. Renal excretion, facilitated by the kidneys, plays a central role in eliminating water-soluble drugs and their metabolites. The glomerular filtration, tubular secretion, and tubular reabsorption processes collectively contribute to the overall renal excretion of drugs [33]. Additionally, hepatic metabolism, involving enzymatic transformations in the liver, leads to the formation of metabolites that are often more hydrophilic and readily excreted by the kidneys. Understanding the biopharmaceutics of drug excretion is crucial for optimizing drug dosages, predicting drug interactions, and ensuring the efficacy and safety of pharmaceutical interventions. Moreover, this knowledge is essential in the development of new drugs and therapeutic strategies aimed at enhancing drug elimination or minimizing undesirable side effects related to drug accumulation [32].

## 14.6 Penicillin Pharmaceutics

The stability and oral absorption of penicillins (refer to Chap. 3) vary due to factors such as their resistance to gastric acid and structure [34]. Most penicillins, except for penicillin G, methicillin, and carbenicillin, are relatively resistant to destruction by gastric acid, but this does not guarantee good oral absorbability. Only 30 to 50% of most penicillins taken orally enter the systemic circulation, with amoxicillin being an exception [34].

Penicillin absorption relies on passive migration across the intestinal mucosa. Penicillins are largely ionized in the intestinal lumen due to their pK values, despite being relatively insoluble in lipids [35]. The affinity of the molecule for the mucosal surface and resistance to acid degradation are significant factors in their absorbability [36]. Food in the stomach can delay and reduce the absorption of most penicillins, except for some, like phenoxymethyl penicillin, ampicillin, and amoxicillin [34].

Serum levels of penicillins after oral administration vary widely due to multiple influencing factors. Notably, the degree of absorption is not solely determined by high-serum concentrations, as protein binding, biotransformation, and excretion also play a role [37]. The type of penicillin, such as isoxazolyl penicillins, can affect serum levels, but differences in free drug concentrations are minimal [34].

Penicillins are well distributed in nonspecialized body fluids and organs, but access to certain sites like the central nervous system, eye, and prostate is challenging due to lipid barriers and active transport pumps for organic anions [38]. Inflammation can reduce these barriers [39,40]. Non-caseous abscesses and synovial fluid are sites with good penicillin penetration [35]. Penicillins are also secreted into bile [41], but this route is less significant in eliminating most penicillins in patients with normal kidney function. However, in patients with kidney issues, such as azotemia, this route can impact drug elimination [34].

### 14.6.1 Bioavailability of Penicillin

Penicillin V exhibits a bioavailability of approximately 65% following its passage through the acidic environment of the stomach. To ensure its effectiveness, it is recommended to administer Penicillin V to a fasting patient, as it tends to degrade in the presence of stomach acid. The typical dosage of Penicillin V varies, ranging from 125 mg to 500 mg, to be taken every 6 to 8 hours, depending on the clinical indication and the patient's weight [42].

### 14.6.2 Bioequivalence of Penicillin

A bioequivalence study was conducted on three distinct penicillin/dihydrostreptomycin combination products for intramuscular administration in dairy calves. The investigation involved analyzing plasma concentrations of penicillin and dihydrostreptomycin, along with creatine phosphokinase concentrations, over a 72-hour period post-drug administration. Results indicated significant variations in the pharmacokinetics of penicillin among the tested products. While the extent of absorption was similar, one product exhibited a notably slower release from the injection site. However, except for the AUC, the 90% confidence intervals for these parameters fell outside the acceptable range of 0.80–1.20, indicating non-bioequivalence in penicillin absorption rate. Similarly, bioequivalence was not established for dihydrostreptomycin, with 90% confidence intervals for $C_{max}$, $t_{max}$, and MRT exceeding the acceptable range. Notably, the product with the slowest penicillin release caused more severe tissue damage, as evidenced by elevated plasma creatine phosphokinase concentrations. Comparing these findings with a previous rabbit study suggested rabbits as a potentially suitable animal model for bioequivalence studies involving penicillin/dihydrostreptomycin combinations, potentially replacing larger animals like calves [43].

## 14.7 Vancomycin Pharmaceutics

Vancomycin (refer to Chap. 4) is frequently delivered via intravenous or oral routes, and there is limited information on intrathecal use. While intramuscular injection of vancomycin is known to cause considerable pain, intravenous administration is preferred for most systemic infections due to its efficacy. When orally administered, vancomycin tends to remain predominantly in the gastrointestinal tract with minimal absorption, a characteristic observed in patients with both normal and impaired renal function [44].

Intraperitoneal administration results in good systemic absorption, making it a potential option for patients with chronic renal failure. Intrathecal administration has not been extensively studied but is believed to have minimal impact on serum levels [44].

Vancomycin undergoes primarily renal excretion with minimal metabolism. Although there might be some extrarenal excretion, potentially hepatic, it is not a prominent factor in most patients. Nearly the entire administered dose of vancomycin can be retrieved in the urine of normal subjects. The primary mechanism for renal excretion is glomerular filtration [44].

During cardiopulmonary bypass, vancomycin is not cleared from the serum, but there is a significant drop in serum concentrations upon initiating the bypass. Therefore, a preoperative dose is required to maintain adequate serum levels for prophylactic use during cardiac surgery [44].

### 14.7.1 Bioavailability of Vancomycin

The bioavailability of oral vancomycin is below 10% [17].

### 14.7.2 Bioequivalence of Vancomycin

There is no requirement for generic intravenous antibiotics to demonstrate therapeutic equivalence with the original product, as equivalence is assumed based on pharmaceutical similarity. To scrutinize these assumptions, a study compared three generic versions of vancomycin with the original product. The investigation evaluated the concentration and efficacy of the active pharmaceutical ingredient using various methods, including microbiological assays, pharmacokinetics in infected mice, antibacterial effects, and pharmacodynamics against *Staphylococcus aureus*. The findings indicated that the generic vancomycin versions were comparable to the original concerning concentration, potency, protein binding, and in vitro antibacterial effects. However, in in vivo testing, the generic products proved ineffective against *S. aureus*, unlike the original product, which exhibited the expected bactericidal efficacy. This analysis suggests that the generic vancomycin versions may contain components in their formulations leading to antagonistic actions, affecting their in vivo efficacy. In conclusion, pharmaceutical equivalence does not necessarily ensure therapeutic equivalence for vancomycin, and generic versions may exhibit complex interactions within their formulations that impact their effectiveness [45].

## 14.8 AMP Pharmaceutics

The pharmacokinetics (PK) and pharmacodynamics (PD) principles in determining the response to antimicrobial peptides, or AMPs (refer to Chap. 5) offer valuable insights into dose regimens for clinical use.

Research conducted by Dosler and colleagues has showcased the in vitro activities of AMPs (Antimicrobial Peptides), both individually and in conjunction with conventional antibiotics, against MRSA (Methicillin-Resistant Staphylococcus Aureus) biofilms. The findings indicated that AMPs enhance the pharmacokinetic efficacy of antibiotics, suggesting a promising approach for enhanced treatment strategies [46].

In a separate investigation conducted by Schmidt and collaborators, it was demonstrated that AMPs Onc72 and Onc112 achieve rapid distribution to various organs following intravenous and intraperitoneal administration. This phenomenon elucidates their heightened in vivo effectiveness, especially in urinary tract infections [47]. Yet, to ascertain the exact correlation between dose, exposure, and response, translational PK/PD modeling and simulation are imperative. PK/PD modeling aids in comprehending the complex interactions involving the specific AMP, bacterial attributes, and the host's response. This comprehension facilitates the optimization of dosing regimens, considering factors such as bacterial eradication, potential side effects, and resistance [48].

Importantly, AMPs exhibit distinct effects on growing bacterial populations compared to antibiotics, particularly from a PD perspective. Studies by Yu and colleagues have indicated that AMPs have a lower likelihood of resistance development due to differences in PD and mutagenic properties compared to antibiotics [49, 50]. Although further reason with diverse AMPs is necessary to establish generalizable PK/PD characteristics, the existing data strongly indicates that AMPs exhibit notable distinctions from antibiotics in terms of both PD and mutagenic properties. This distinction positions AMPs as promising candidates for addressing the evolution of resistance. 15.5.3.2 Bioavailability of AMPs: Typically, oral peptide bioavailability is limited to less than 1–2% due to gastrointestinal degradation and low permeability [51].

## 14.9 Quinolone Pharmaceutics

Fluoroquinolones (refer to Chap. 6) are a group of antibiotics known for their rapid absorption when administered orally. The time it takes to reach the maximum concentration in the bloodstream ($t_{max}$) after oral administration typically ranges from 0.5 to 3.0 hours [52]. Some specific fluoroquinolones like lomefloxacin and ciprofloxacin achieve their peak concentrations within 1–2 hours, while there can be variations in the maximum plasma concentrations based on the dose [53].

As an example, following a 400 mg oral dose of norfloxacin, the $C_{max}$ falls within the range of 1.4–1.6 mg/L. However, this bioavailability diminishes with escalating doses, averaging approximately 70% [54]. Likewise, ciprofloxacin can attain a $C_{max}$ of 2.5 mg/L after a 500 mg dose, although variations in bioavailability can arise due to the use of different dosage forms of the drug [55].

In contrast, fleroxacin achieves an average $C_{max}$ of 5–6 mg/L following a single 400 mg dose, while pefloxacin reaches a $C_{max}$ of 6.0–6.5 mg/L after a 600 mg dose. Ofloxacin also attains a higher mean $C_{max}$ value of 3.2–5.0 mg/L after a 400 mg dose, exhibiting dose proportionality with increasing oral doses and approaching an absolute bioavailability of 100%. Similarly, lomefloxacin demonstrates a correlation between dose and $C_{max}$ in the range of 100–800 mg following a single-dose oral administration, with a $C_{max}$ of 3.0–5.2 mg/L after a 400 mg dose [56].

The absorption of fluoroquinolones is minimally influenced by food. Specifically, ofloxacin, ciprofloxacin, pefloxacin, and lomefloxacin are not significantly affected by food in terms of absorption. However, the rate of absorption may vary among different quinolones. For instance, food intake can decrease the $C_{max}$ for ofloxacin to 69% and extend $t_{max}$ by 203% compared to the fasting state. In contrast, the impact of food on lomefloxacin absorption is less pronounced, with the AUC reduced to 91–94%, $C_{max}$ decreased to 83–87%, and $t_{max}$ prolonged to 169–172% [53]. The type of meal (standard vs. high fat) does not significantly affect the interaction of food with lomefloxacin absorption [57]. The clinical significance of food effects on quinolones is speculative but may impact efficacy, particularly if $C_{max}$ is significantly reduced.

Accumulation of fluoroquinolones can occur following multiple doses, with the extent of accumulation linked to renal impairment. Some quinolones, like ofloxacin, exhibit a small degree of accumulation of the parent drug, while others, such as enoxacin, pefloxacin, and ciprofloxacin, can accumulate metabolites. Lomefloxacin does not accumulate after multiple doses in healthy individuals, and its $C_{max}$ values approximate those measured after a single dosing [53].

The protein binding of newer fluoroquinolones is relatively modest, measuring around 30% for ciprofloxacin, 20% for ofloxacin, and 10% for lomefloxacin. Moreover, these antibiotics exhibit exceptional and comparable penetration into diverse tissues, with peak concentrations in specific tissues (such as prostatic and gynecologic tissue, bile, liver, gall bladder tissue, and pancreatic fluid) several times higher than those in the serum. Tissue penetration levels, however, vary among different fluoroquinolones, and concentrations in sputum and bronchial secretions also show distinctions [53].

Metabolism and elimination pathways for fluoroquinolones exhibit notable variations. Certain quinolones undergo extensive metabolic biotransformation, resulting in distinctions in total body clearance and elimination half-life. Specifically, pefloxacin exemplifies high metabolic activity, with less than 10% recovered as an unchanged drug in urine [58]. Conversely, ofloxacin experiences almost no metabolic biotransformation, with 70–80% of the dose excreted renally as unchanged drug. Lomefloxacin and fleroxacin demonstrate moderate levels of metabolism. Enoxacin and ciprofloxacin similarly undergo metabolic processes, where hepatic extraction and excretion into the bowel significantly contribute to nonrenal clearance [59].

The elimination half-life varies among fluoroquinolones, with pefloxacin, ofloxacin, lomefloxacin, and ciprofloxacin having longer half-lives, while ciprofloxacin has a relatively short half-life. Norfloxacin falls within the intermediate range of half-life. Metabolites of various degrees of antibacterial activity have been identified for these drugs, influencing their overall pharmacokinetics. About 30% of norfloxacin is recovered unchanged in urine [60, 61].

In summary, fluoroquinolones exhibit rapid oral absorption, with variations in absorption characteristics and bioavailability among different class members. Food has minimal effects on their absorption. Accumulation may occur following multiple doses, particularly for quinolones with metabolites. The extent of protein binding, tissue penetration, and metabolic pathways varies among fluoroquinolones, leading to differences in their elimination half-lives and pharmacokinetics.

### 14.9.1 Quinolone Bioavailability

Quinolones are typically well absorbed when administered orally, with bioavailability ranging from moderate to excellent [62].

## 14.10 Rifampicin Pharmaceutics

Gastric pH plays a significant role in the absorption of rifampicin (refer to Chap. 7) in humans. Acidifying gastric juice with histamine results in serum concentrations that are twice as high as those observed after alkalization with sodium bicarbonate [63]. These findings are consistent with previous research that noted variations in serum rifampicin levels when administered on an empty or full stomach. Based on these studies, it is recommended to administer rifampicin on an empty stomach, as under these conditions, the absorption of rifampicin is both rapid and nearly complete. The so-called first-pass hepatic effect, where the drug passes through the hepatoportal system and enters the bile, is a crucial factor influencing the time course of rifampicin concentrations in the systemic circulation [63].

Regarding metabolism, the primary metabolic derivative of human rifampicin is desacetylrifampicin, which is microbiologically active, albeit less so than the parent drug. This derivative represents the main fraction of bile. Desacetylation of rifampicin likely occurs in the hepatocyte, resulting in a more polar compound that facilitates excretion in bile [63]. A small portion of the antibacterial activity in human urine is represented by formyl rifampicin, which may form spontaneously in the urine, although its metabolic origin is not entirely ruled out [64].

Biliary excretion of rifampicin is evident within the first hour after oral administration, with concentrations reaching a plateau 4 to 5 hours later. Data on biliary excretion from various rifampicin doses supports the hypothesis that the liver's excretory capacity for rifampicin decreases with higher daily doses, as reported by Pechere and Tancrede [64].

### 14.10.1 Bioavailability of Rifampicin

Rifampicin demonstrated an absolute bioavailability of over 86% when oral administration was compared with both 30-minute and 3-hour infusions [65].

### 14.10.2 Bioequivalence of Rifampicin

In a comparative study, the bioavailability of a novel rifampicin formulation, Rifampicine Generic (300 mg capsules), was evaluated against a reference form, Rimactan (300 mg capsules), employing a cross-over design with twelve healthy volunteers. Both formulations were well-tolerated, and no adverse effects were observed. Rifampicin plasma concentrations were analyzed using HPLC in blood samples collected over 10 hours. The pharmacokinetic parameters ($C_{max}$, $t_{max}$, AUC0-10h) demonstrated similarity between the new and reference forms, and statistical analyses affirmed their bioequivalence. Consequently, it was concluded that Rifampicine Generic 300 mg capsules are bioequivalent to Rimactan 300 mg capsules [66].

## 14.11 Tetracycline Pharmaceutics

The absorption of tetracycline antibiotics (refer to Chap. 8) is subject to variability, typically falling within the range of 25–60%. Absorption occurs gradually following oral administration, primarily in the stomach, duodenum, and small intestine. $C_{max}$ typically ranges from 1 to 5 mg/L, with a $t_{max}$ of 2–4 hours, except for demeclocycline, which exhibits a delayed $C_{max}$ at 4–6 hours. Tetracyclines can form insoluble complexes with calcium, magnesium, iron, and aluminum, leading to reduced absorption. Meals rich in protein, fat, and carbohydrates can diminish tetracycline absorption by approximately 50%. The volume of distribution (V) is approximately 1.3–1.7 L/kg, and data on tissue distribution is generally of poor quality, making it challenging to draw definitive conclusions. Protein binding varies among different tetracycline antibiotics [67].

Metabolism is generally limited for tetracycline antibiotics, except for tetracycline, where 5% is excreted as the metabolite Δ-epitetracycline. These drugs are primarily excreted unchanged through renal and biliary routes, with renal elimination (CLR) predominantly associated with glomerular filtration, except for chlortetracycline. Less than 50% of the drugs are excreted in urine, while over 40% are excreted in feces, mainly through biliary elimination. Most drugs exhibit some degree of enterohepatic circulation, with biliary concentrations surpassing blood concentrations by a factor of 5. Serum concentration-time profiles demonstrate a plateau-shaped course, characterized by a slow rise and a slower decline, and serum half-lives ($t_{1/2}$) range from 6 to 17 hours. Serum concentrations increase with higher doses, and there is limited data available on the areas under the serum time curves [67].

Effects on the pharmacokinetics in special groups, such as age, sex, obesity, low body weight, infections, other comorbidities, and liver impairment, are not well understood. The impact of exercise on tetracycline includes increased serum concentrations and reduced renal clearance, although its clinical significance remains uncertain. Renal failure has a notable effect on tetracycline elimination but has minimal impact on chlortetracycline, maintaining a comparable serum half-life in patients with chronic renal failure as in those with normal renal function [67].

### 14.11.1 Tetracycline Bioavailability

The bioavailability of the substance is below 40% when administered through intramuscular injection, 100% when given intravenously, and ranges from 60–80% when taken orally (in fasting adults) [68].

### 14.11.2 Tetracycline Bioequivalence

In this investigation, the bioequivalence of two long-acting oxytetracycline (OTC) formulations, Terramycin LA (Pfizer) and Cyamicin LA (Fort Dodge Saude Animal), was assessed in clinically healthy bovines. Both formulations were intramuscularly administered at 20 mg OTC/kg, and plasma samples were analyzed using high-pressure liquid chromatography. Bioavailability parameters ($C_{max}$, $AUC_{0\rightarrow\infty}$) were compared using analysis of variance and 90% confidence interval tests, while nonparametric tests were employed for $t_{max}$. Although $AUC_{0\rightarrow\infty}$ and $t_{max}$ values showed no significant differences, the mean $C_{max}$ of the test product differed significantly from the reference (8.73 ±3.66 μg/mL versus 10.43 ±3.84 μg/mL). The 90% confidence intervals for $AUC_{0\rightarrow\infty}$ and $t_{max}$ fell within the 80–125% range, but for $C_{max}$, it extended beyond this range. Consequently, it was concluded that the $C_{max}$ of the test product deviates by more than 20% from that of the reference, indicating a lack of bioequivalence between the test OTC and the reference formulation [69].

## 14.12 Streptomycin Pharmaceutics

Streptomycin (refer to Chap. 9), a potent antibiotic, exhibits promising therapeutic potential in treating experimental infections caused by gram-negative bacteria and *Mycobacterium tuberculosis*. Despite limited clinical reports on human applications, ongoing studies aim to enhance our understanding of streptomycin's effectiveness as production escalates. Administration routes, including intravenous, intramuscular, subcutaneous, and intrathecal, have been explored, shedding light on the drug's stability and persistence in various bodily compartments. Noteworthy findings include variations in serum concentrations based on administration routes, slower urinary excretion compared to penicillin, and incomplete absorption from the subarachnoid space following intrathecal injection. These insights contribute valuable information to the broader understanding of streptomycin's pharmacokinetics and underscore its potential significance in clinical therapeutics [70].

### 14.12.1 Streptomycin Bioavailability

Streptomycin's bioavailability is 84 to 88% [71].

### 14.12.2 Streptomycin Bioequivalence

The above study [71] aimed to assess the comparative bioequivalence of Estreptovall and Nilestrept in healthy broiler chickens following intramuscular (IM) injection of a 25 mg streptomycin base/kg.b.wt. dose for each product. The experiment involved 24 broiler chickens divided into two groups, with the first group focusing on

Estreptovall's pharmacokinetics and the second on Nilestrept's. Blood samples were collected before and at various intervals up to 24 hours after a single IM injection. The disposition kinetics analysis revealed that both Estreptovall and Nilestrept reached maximum blood concentrations ($C_{max}$) of 25.75 and 23.84 μg/ml, respectively, with peak times ($t_{max}$) of 2.50 and 2.51 hours. The calculated ratios of $C_{max}$, $AUC_{0\rightarrow 24}$, and $AUC_{0\rightarrow \infty}$ (T/R for Nilestrept compared to Estreptovall were 0.93, 0.92, and 0.92, respectively), falling within the bioequivalence acceptance range. Consequently, the study concludes that Nilestrept is bioequivalent to Estreptovall, suggesting interchangeability regarding streptomycin pharmacokinetics in broiler chickens [72].

## 14.13 Chloramphenicol Pharmaceutics

Chloramphenicol (refer to Chap. 10), in its various forms, is subject to differences in absorption and bioavailability due to particle size. Smaller particle sizes lead to faster absorption rates, but the extent of absorption remains similar to products with larger particles. These principles apply to other drugs as well. Bioavailability of chloramphenicol base is estimated through urinary recovery, generally ranging from 76% to 93%. Peak plasma concentrations occur between 0.5 and 6 hours after administration [73].

Chloramphenicol palmitate, in contrast, does not undergo direct absorption. Instead, it undergoes hydrolysis in the small intestine to produce free chloramphenicol. The rate of hydrolysis is associated with particle size. The bioavailability of chloramphenicol, determined by urinary recovery, is approximately 80% when administered as a suspension of chloramphenicol palmitate. Peak plasma concentrations are observed about 2–3 hours after oral administration, with elevated peaks achieved when administered in a fasting state [73].

Chloramphenicol succinate is used for parenteral administration and is considered a prodrug. The conversion from succinate to active chloramphenicol is often incomplete, as renal excretion of intact chloramphenicol succinate reduces the amount available for conversion. The time to reach peak plasma concentrations varies widely, ranging from 18 minutes to 3 hours [73].

Chloramphenicol is extensively distributed throughout various tissues and body fluids, including the brain, heart, lungs, kidneys, liver, spleen, vitreous humor, breast milk, CSF, and more. It crosses the placenta [73].

The protein binding of chloramphenicol is around 53–66%, primarily with albumin. The unbound fraction is considered the active form, and an increased unbound fraction can lead to higher pharmacological activity. In CSF, higher antibacterial activity was observed, despite lower concentrations than in the serum [73].

Chloramphenicol is mainly eliminated through metabolism to inactive products, with the principal metabolite being a glucuronide conjugate excreted in the urine. Some hydrolysis products have been identified. There is no evidence of concentration-dependent metabolism. Renal excretion involves glomerular filtration, with approximately 5–15% of unconjugated chloramphenicol being excreted unchanged in the urine. Renal elimination of chloramphenicol succinate may involve active tubular secretion, but details vary [73]. Extracorporeal elimination methods, such as hemodialysis, can be effective for removing chloramphenicol in overdose situations. Peritoneal dialysis is not as effective for removal. In cases of severe chloramphenicol intoxication, exchange transfusions or charcoal hemoperfusion may be considered for rapid removal of the drug, but these treatments should not be considered routine and need further investigation [73].

### 14.13.1 Chloramphenicol Bioavailability

Chloramphenicol is swiftly and fully absorbed from the gastrointestinal tract after oral administration, with a determined bioavailability of 80% [74].

### 14.13.2 Chloramphenicol Bioequivalence

In studies involving cats, it was observed that chloramphenicol tablets and chloramphenicol palmitate suspension were bioinequivalent in fasted conditions, with the liquid formulation exhibiting slower and reduced systemic drug availability. However, when cats were fed ad libitum, the availability from the suspension improved and became like that of tablets. The suboptimal performance of the suspension could pose a risk of therapeutic failure in sick cats not eating. This research highlights the influence of ingesta on bioavailability, showcasing varied effects with different drug formulations. Injectable chloramphenicol preparations were also found to be bioinequivalent after intramuscular use in cats, with significant differences in $C_{max}$ and AUC values observed between chloramphenicol sodium succinate solution and chloramphenicol dissolved in methylpyrrolidone or an aqueous suspension of chloramphenicol. While some studies indicated bioequivalence in capsules and tablets for cats and fasted greyhounds, discrepancies were found in dogs among injectable products and oral preparations [75].

## 14.14 Antimetabolite Pharmaceutics

Antimetabolites (refer to Chap. 11) play a crucial role in cancer chemotherapy, with drugs like Ara-C, thiopurines, and MTX used for childhood and adult leukemia, and new adenosine analogs showing potential against conditions like hairy cell leukemia and malignant lymphomas. Methotrexate and 5-fluorouracil (5FU) are employed for various solid malignancies. Recent advancements in the clinical pharmacology of antimetabolites have unveiled the relationship between dose, plasma concentrations, clearance, toxicity, and antitumor effects. For example, adaptive control of 5FU administration can reduce its toxicity. Pharmacogenetics, like 6MP and 5FU, may aid in identifying patients at higher risk of toxicity. Some evidence exists for identifying populations at risk of nonresponse to Ara-C [76].

Moreover, there is substantial evidence of the intracellular (intratumor) metabolism of most antimetabolites, which allows for the identification of potential treatment responders. Accumulation of active metabolites (e.g., ara-CTP, thioguanine nucleotides, FdUMP, MTX-polyglutamates) and the inhibition of target enzymes (e.g., thymidylate synthase) have laid the foundation for biochemical modulation. This approach involves the specific manipulation of the drug's intracellular metabolism. Future advancements in molecular biology, biochemistry, cell biology, and immunology are expected to enhance the identification of resistant patients, enabling the specific modulation of drug metabolism in tumor cells. Biochemical modulation has already yielded significant treatment improvements and is a fundamental aspect of cancer chemotherapy. As new antimetabolites emerge, biochemical modulation, often in combination with other drugs or biologicals, will continue to be a major strategy for enhancing cancer treatment [77].

## 14.15 MAI Pharmaceutics

The biopharmaceutics of mycolic acid inhibitors (MAIs) represent a critical area of study in the context of tuberculosis (TB) treatment. Mycolic acids are essential components of the mycobacterial cell wall, playing a pivotal role in its structural integrity and impermeability. Inhibitors targeting mycolic acid biosynthesis form a cornerstone in the development of anti-TB drugs. The biopharmaceutical aspects encompass drug absorption, distribution, metabolism, and excretion, influencing their therapeutic efficacy. Understanding the pharmacokinetics of mycolic acid inhibitors is vital for optimizing dosage regimens, enhancing drug delivery, and minimizing adverse effects. Moreover, as mycobacteria often reside within macrophages, the formulation and delivery systems must consider intracellular drug penetration. Advances in biopharmaceutical research on mycolic acid inhibitors contribute significantly to refining treatment strategies for TB, a global health concern. This knowledge aids in the development of more effective and patient-friendly formulations, ultimately bolstering the arsenal against tuberculosis [78].

## 14.16 Case Studies

Case studies hold significant importance in the realm of biopharmaceutics as invaluable tools for delving into the real-world application and outcomes of pharmaceutical interventions. These in-depth analyses of individual or group experiences provide a nuanced understanding of how biopharmaceuticals perform in diverse clinical scenarios, shedding light on factors such as patient variability, treatment responses, and potential adverse effects. Case studies not only complement data derived from controlled clinical trials but also offer valuable insights into the practical challenges and successes encountered in biopharmaceutical use, contributing essential knowledge for clinicians, researchers, and regulators in optimizing treatment strategies and ensuring patient safety.

### 14.16.1 Penicillin

In a case study by Rammelkamp et al., the materials and methods employed in investigating the pharmacokinetics of penicillins are detailed. The study involved normal volunteers and ward patients, primarily suffering from localized infections. Penicillin, in the form of the sodium salt, was administered through various routes, including oral, intravenous, intramuscular, rectal, and others. The concentrations of penicillin in blood plasma and urine were measured at different intervals. The study revealed rapid rise and fall patterns in serum concentrations after intravenous administration, contrasting with delayed appearances and prolonged durations for intramuscular and subcutaneous injections. Additionally, the research explored the effects of renal function on penicillin excretion, indicating a prolonged presence in subjects with renal failure. The distribution of penicillin between blood plasma and erythrocytes was examined, suggesting minimal penetration of red cells. The findings underscored the importance of considering infection type and location in determining the route and dosage of penicillin administration for effective therapy [79].

### 14.16.2 Streptomycin

In a case study on streptomycin by Anderson et al., the materials and methods involved adult ward patients with no renal impairment. Streptomycin, supplied by Merck and Company, was used in concentrations ranging from 50,000 to 150,000 units per cubic centimeter for various administrations. The drug's stability was ensured by storing solutions at 5°C. Blood samples, assayed using the cup-plate method, were taken under sterile conditions. Urinary excretion studies were conducted in male patients, storing samples at 5°C. The assay method proved satisfactory for concentrations up to 20 units per cubic centimeter. Pharmacologic studies included oral, intravenous, and intramuscular administration. Streptomycin's absorption, serum concentrations, and urinary excretion were investigated. The study also explored streptomycin's diffusion into spinal fluid. The case reports detailed streptomycin therapy in patients with typhoid fever and pyelonephritis, highlighting clinical responses and potential toxicities. The study concluded with insights into streptomycin's absorption, excretion, and potential therapeutic applications, emphasizing the need for careful administration to manage discomfort and potential adverse reactions [70].

### 14.16.3 Rifampicin

In the biopharmaceutical analysis of rifampicin for newborns and infants, proportional doses based on mg/kg body weight result in serum levels generally lower than those observed in adults. This discrepancy, especially pronounced in infants, is attributed to larger total body water compartments. Newborns exhibit less efficient drug elimination, likely through bile, leading to drug accumulation with repeated administration. In infants, [80] suggests a half-life of 2.55±0.98 hours, indicating that doses higher than 10mg/kg, possibly based on body surface area, are needed, cautioning against exceeding this dosage in newborns. For patients with impaired liver function, rifampicin concentrations rise, and its half-life significantly increases. Cirrhotic patients demonstrate a prolonged half-life (5.42±0.55 hours) compared to controls (2.80±0.22 hours). Liver disease type or acuteness does not affect this finding, with serum concentrations consistently higher in liver disease. In patients with impaired kidney function, renal clearance of rifampicin diminishes, attributed to a potential 75% binding to serum proteins. Despite lower-than-expected clearance values, rifampicin can be administered at normal therapeutic doses to patients with severe renal impairment. The serum level curve in renal impairment shows progressively higher and prolonged values, particularly after 4 hours post-administration, and remains evident at 24 hours. Dialysis procedures impact rifampicin levels, with peritoneal dialysis demonstrating dialyzability, while hemodialysis results in a sharp decrease toward normal values after 4 hours [63].

## References


1. Balick MJ, Cox PA (2020) Plants, people, and culture: the science of ethnobotany. Garland Science
2. Yapijakis C (2009) Hippocrates of Kos, the father of clinical medicine, and Asclepiades of Bithynia, the father of molecular medicine. In vivo 23(4):507–514
3. Chen S, Chen Q, Askool YS, Xu L (2023) Textual research on Dioscorides and De Materia Medica. Chinese Med 14(3):208–219
4. Abbasi MUR, Rasool S, Kashan S, Rehman ZU, Athar S, Iftikhar I (2023) Medicine in the medieval Islamic world, innovation and public policy and historical rulers perspective. Al-Qanṭara 9(3):179–186
5. Rang HP (2006) The receptor concept: pharmacology's big idea. B J Pharmacol 147(S1):S9–S16
6. Borchers AT, et al. (2007) The history and contemporary challenges of the US Food and Drug Administration. Clinical therapeutics 29(1):1–16
7. Todorović Z, Vučković S, Divac N (2022) Pharmacology, from Rudolf Buchheim to Arnold Holste: the founding of the Institute of Pharmacology at the Faculty of Medicine, University of Belgrade. Scripta Medica 53(1):82–88
8. Levy G (1998) Predicting effective drug concentrations for individual patients: determinants of pharmacodynamic variability. Clin Pharmacokinet 34(4):323–333
9. Panchagnula R, Thomas NS (2000) Biopharmaceutics and pharmacokinetics in drug research. Int J Pharmaceut 201(2):131–150
10. Basanta Kumar Reddy B, Karunakar A (2011) Biopharmaceutics classification system: a regulatory approach. Dissolution Technol 18(1):31–37

11. Dressman JB, Amidon GL, Fleisher D (1985) Absorption potential: estimating the fraction absorbed for orally administered compounds. J Pharmaceut Sci 74(5):588–589
12. Sinko PJ, Leesman GD, Amidon GL (1991) Predicting fraction dose absorbed in humans using a macroscopic mass balance approach. Pharmaceut Res 8:979–988
13. Shah VP, Amidon GL, Lennernas H, Crison JR (1995) A theoretical basis for a biopharmaceutic drug classification: The correlation of in vitro drug product dissolution and in vivo bioavailability. Pharm Res 12:413–420—Backstory of BCS. AAPS J 16:894–898 (2014)
14. Oh D-M, Curl RL, Amidon GL (1993) Estimating the fraction dose absorbed from suspensions of poorly soluble compounds in humans: a mathematical model. Pharmaceut Res 10:264–270
15. Rajesh D (2015) The need of a uniform drug classification in text books of pharmacology. Ind J Pharmacol 47(6):695–696
16. Milani DAQ, Davis DD (2020) Pain management medications. StatPearls Publishing
17. Patel S, Preuss CV, Bernice F (2017) Vancomycin. StatPearls Publishing
18. Khalil H, Zeltser R (2022) Antihypertensive medications. In: StatPearls [Internet]. StatPearls Publishing
19. Gosmanov AR, Gosmanova EO, Dillard-Cannon E (2014) Management of adult diabetic ketoacidosis. Diabetes, metabolic syndrome and obesity: targets and therapy, pp. 255–264
20. Yalkowsky SH (1981) Solubility and solubilization of nonelectrolites. Drugs Pharm Sci 12:1–14
21. Bohacek RS, McMartin C, Guida WC (1996) The art and practice of structure-based drug design: a molecular modeling perspective. Med Res Rev 16(1):3–50
22. Vacca JP, Guare JP, Desolms SJ, Sanders WM, Giuliani EA, Young SD, Darke PL, Sigal IS, Schleif WA (1991) L-687,908, a potent hydroxyethylene containing HIV protease inhibitor. J Med Chem 34(3):1225–1228
23. Stella VJ, Martodihardjo S, Terada K, Rao VM (1998) Some relationships between the physical properties of various 3-acyloxymethyl prodrugs of phenytoin to structure: Potential in vivo performance implications. J Pharmaceut Sci 87(10):1235–1241
24. Müller BW, Brauns U (1985) Solubilization of drugs by modified $\beta$-cyclodextrins. Int J Pharmaceut 26(1-2):77–88
25. Smith RN, Hansch C, Ames MM (1975) Selection of a reference partitioning system for drug design work. J Pharmaceut Sci 64(4):599–606
26. Smith DA, Jones BC, Walker DK (1996) Design of drugs involving the concepts and theories of drug metabolism and pharmacokinetics. Med Res Rev 16(3):243–266
27. Barton P, Davis AM, Webborn PJH, McCarthy DJ (1997) Drug-phospholipid interactions. 2. predicting the sites of drug distribution using n-octanol/water and membrane/water distribution coefficients. J Pharmaceut Sci 86(9):1034–1039
28. Abraham MH, Chadha HS, Mitchell RC (1994) Hydrogen bonding. 33. factors that influence the distribution of solutes between blood and brain. J Pharmaceut Sci 83(9):1257–1268
29. Toon S, Rowland M (1983) Structure-pharmacokinetic relationships among the barbiturates in the rat. J Pharmacol Exp Therapeut 225(3):752–763
30. Martin Y (1971) Influence of hydrophobic character on the relative rate of oxidation of drugs by rat liver microsomes. J Med Chem 14(9):777–779
31. Kleinert HD, Rosenberg SH, Baker WR, Stein HH, Klinghofer V, Barlow J, Spina K, Polakowski J, Kovar P, Cohen J, et al. (1992) Discovery of a peptide-based renin inhibitor with oral bioavailability and efficacy. Science 257(5078):1940–1943
32. Alsanosi SMM, Skiffington C, Padmanabhan S (2014) Pharmacokinetic pharmacogenomics, pp 341–364. Academic Press, London
33. Yang Y, Zhao Y, Yu A, Sun D, Yu L (2017) Oral drug absorption: Evaluation and prediction. In: Developing solid oral dosage forms, pp 331–354. Elsevier
34. Barza M, Weinstein L (1976) Pharmacokinetics of the penicillins in man. Clin Pharmacokinet 1(4):297–308
35. Howell A, Sutherland R, Rolinson GN (1972) Effect of protein binding on levels of ampicillin and cloxacillin in synovial fluid. Clin Pharmacol Therapeut 13(5part1):724–732

36. Rollo IM (1972) Physiological disposition of some semisynthetic penicillins. Can J Physiol Pharmacol 50(10):986–998
37. McCarthy CG, Finland M, Wilcox C, Yarrows JH (1960) Absorption and excretion of four penicillins: penicillin g, penicillin v, phenethicillin and phenylmercaptomethyl penicillin. New Engl J Med 263(7):315–326
38. Hogben CAM (1971) Biological membranes and their passage by drugs. In: Concepts in biochemical pharmacology: part 1, pp 1–8. Springer
39. Thrupp LD, Leedom JM, Ivler D, Wehrle PF, Portnoy B, Mathies AW (1965) Ampicillin levels in the cerebrospinal fluid during treatment of bacterial meningitis. Antimicrobial Agents Chemotherapy 5:206–213
40. Taber LH, Yow MD, George Nieberg F (1967) The penetration of broad-spectrum antibiotics into the cerebrospinal fxuid. Ann New York Acad Sci 145(2):473–481
41. Smith RL (1971) Excretion of drugs in bile. In: Concepts in biochemical pharmacology: part 1, pp 354–389. Springer
42. Yip DW, Gerriets V (2020) Penicillin
43. Groen K, Mevius DJ, Fauw DP-D, De Neeling AJ, Vulto AG (1996) Bioequivalence study in calves of three commercial penicillin/dihydrostreptomycin fixed combination products for intramuscular injection. J Veterinary Pharmacol Therapeut 19(5):370–375
44. Moellering RC Jr. (1984) Pharmacokinetics of vancomycin. J Antimicrobial Chemotherapy 14(suppl_D):43–52
45. Vesga O, Agudelo M, Salazar BE, Rodriguez CA, Zuluaga AF (2010) Generic vancomycin products fail in vivo despite being pharmaceutical equivalents of the innovator. Antimicrobial Agents Chemotherapy 54(8):3271–3279
46. Dosler S, Mataraci E (2013) In vitro pharmacokinetics of antimicrobial cationic peptides alone and in combination with antibiotics against methicillin resistant staphylococcus aureus biofilms. Peptides 49:53–58
47. Schmidt R, Ostorházi E, Wende E, Knappe D, Hoffmann R (2016) Pharmacokinetics and in vivo efficacy of optimized oncocin derivatives. J Antimicrobial Chemotherapy 71(4):1003–1011
48. Rathi C, Lee RE, Meibohm B (2016) Translational pk/pd of anti-infective therapeutics. Drug Disc Today Technol 21:41–49
49. Yu G, Baeder DY, Regoes RR, Rolff J (2016) Combination effects of antimicrobial peptides. Antimicrobial Agents Chemotherapy 60(3):1717–1724
50. Yu G, Baeder DY, Regoes RR, Rolff J (2018) Predicting drug resistance evolution: insights from antimicrobial peptides and antibiotics. Proc Roy Soc B Biol Sci 285(1874):20172687
51. Han Y, Gao Z, Chen L, Kang L, Huang W, Jin M, Wang Q, Bae YH (2019) Multifunctional oral delivery systems for enhanced bioavailability of therapeutic peptides/proteins. Acta Pharmaceutica Sinica B 9(5):902–922
52. Bergan T, Delin C, Johansen S, Kolstad IM, Nord CE, Thorsteinsson SB (1986) Pharmacokinetics of ciprofloxacin and effect of repeated dosage on salivary and fecal microflora. Antimicrobial Agents Chemotherapy 29(2):298–302
53. Robson RA (1992) Quinolone pharmacokinetics. Int J Antimicrobial Agents 2(1):3–10
54. Holmes B, Brogden RN, Richards DM (1985) Norfloxacin: a review of its antibacterial activity, pharmacokinetic properties and therapeutic use. Drugs 30:482–513
55. Davis RL, Koup JR, Williams-Warren J, Weber A, Smith AL (1985) Pharmacokinetics of three oral formulations of ciprofloxacin. Antimicrobial Agents Chemotherapy 28(1):74–77
56. Hooper WD, Dickinson RG, Eadie MJ (1990) Effect of food on absorption of lomefloxacin. Antimicrobial Agents Chemotherapy 34(9):1797–1799
57. Lode H, Höffken G, Olschewski P, Sievers B, Kirch A, Borner K, Koeppe P (1987) Pharmacokinetics of ofloxacin after parenteral and oral administration. Antimicrobial Agents Chemotherapy 31(9):1338–1342
58. Montay G, Goueffon Y, Roquet F (1984) Absorption, distribution, metabolic fate, and elimination of pefloxacin mesylate in mice, rats, dogs, monkeys, and humans. Antimicrobial Agents Chemotherapy 25(4):463–472

59. Bury RW, Becker GJ, Kincaid-Smith PS, Moulds RFW, Whitworth JA (1987) Elimination of enoxacin in renal disease. Clin Pharmacol Therapeut 41(4):434–438
60. Fillastre JP, Leroy A, Moulin B, Dhib M, Borsa-Lebas F, Humbert G (1990) Pharmacokinetics of quinolones in renal insufficiency. J Antimicrobial Chemotherapy 26(suppl_B):51–60
61. Yang X, Yousef AE (2018) Antimicrobial peptides produced by Brevibacillus spp.: structure, classification and bioactivity: a mini review. World J Microbiol Biotechnol 34:1–10
62. Oliphant CM, Green GM (2002) Quinolones: a comprehensive review. Am Family Physician 65(3):455–465
63. Acocella G (1978) Clinical pharmacokinetics of rifampicin. Clin Pharmacokinet 3:108–127
64. Nakagawa H, Sunahara S (1975) Glucuronidation and desacetylation in the metabolism of rifampicin in man. In: Twenty-third International Tuberculosis Conference, Mexico City
65. Mariappan TT, Singh S, Pandey R, Khuller GK (2005) Determination of absolute bioavailability of rifampicin by varying the mode of intravenous administration and the time of sampling. Clin Res Regulat Affairs 22(3-4):119–128
66. Chouchane N, Barre J, Toumi A, Tillement JP, Benakis A (1995) Bioequivalence study of two pharmaceutical forms of rifampicin capsules in man. Eur J Drug Metabolism Pharmacokinet 20:315–320
67. Agwuh KN, MacGowan A (2006) Pharmacokinetics and pharmacodynamics of the tetracyclines including glycylcyclines. J Antimicrobial Chemotherapy 58(2):256–265
68. Welling PG, Koch PA, Lau CC, Craig WA (1977) Bioavailability of tetracycline and doxycycline in fasted and nonfasted subjects. Antimicrobial Agents Chemotherapy 11(3):462–469
69. Mestorino N, Marchetti ML, Lucas MF, Modamio P, Zeinsteger P, Lastra CF, Segarra I, Mariño EL (2016) Bioequivalence study of two long-acting formulations of oxytetracycline following intramuscular administration in bovines. Front Veterinary Sci 3:50
70. Anderson DG, Jewell M (1945) The absorption, excretion and toxicity of streptomycin in man. New Engl J Med 233(17):485–491
71. Zhu M, Burman WJ, Jaresko GS, Berning SE, Jelliffe RW, Peloquin CA (2001) Population pharmacokinetics of intravenous and intramuscular streptomycin in patients with tuberculosis. Pharmacotherapy J Hum Pharmacol Drug Therapy 21(9):1037–1045
72. El-Komy A, Aboubakr M (2023) Bioequivalence study of two streptomycin formulations (Estreptovall and Nilestrept) in broiler chickens. Int J Adv Res (IJAR) 11(10):1–6
73. Ambrose PJ (1984) Clinical pharmacokinetics of chloramphenicol and chloramphenicol succinate. Clin Pharmacokinet 9(3):222–238
74. Kauffman RE, Thirumoorthi MC, Buckley JA, Aravind MK, Dajani AS (1981) Relative bioavailability of intravenous chloramphenicol succinate and oral chloramphenicol palmitate in infants and children. J Pediatr 99(6):963–967
75. Watson ADJ (1992) Bioavailability and bioinequivalence of drug formulations in small animals. J Veterinary Pharmacol Therapeut 15(2):151–159
76. Peters GJ, Schornagel JH, Milano GA (1993) Clinical pharmacokinetics of anti-metabolites. Cancer Surv 17:123–156
77. Wilkins MR, Crowston JG, Cordeiro MF, Khaw PT (1997) Antimetabolites. In: Seminars in ophthalmology, vol 12, pp 143–150. Taylor & Francis
78. Schroeder EK, Norberto de Souza O, Santos DS, Blanchard JS, Basso LA (2002) Drugs that inhibit mycolic acid biosynthesis in mycobacterium tuberculosis. Current Pharmaceut Botechnol 3(3):197–225
79. Rammelkamp CH, Keefer CS, et al. (1943) The absorption, excretion, and distribution of penicillin. J Clin Investigat 22(3):425–437
80. Krauer B, Spring P, Dettli, L (1968) Zur pharmakokinetik der sulfonamide in ersten lebensjahr. Pharmacologia Clinica 1:47–53

MIX
Papier aus verantwortungsvollen Quellen
Paper from responsible sources
FSC® C105338

If you have any concerns about our products,
you can contact us on
**ProductSafety@springernature.com**

In case Publisher is established outside the EU,
the EU authorized representative is:
**Springer Nature Customer Service Center GmbH**
**Europaplatz 3, 69115 Heidelberg, Germany**

Printed by Libri Plureos GmbH
in Hamburg, Germany